Lectin-Free Cookbook:

Delightful & Delicious Lectin-Free Recipes

Table of Contents

written consent and can in no way be considered an
endorsement from the trademark holder.

Introduction

The lectin-free diet is one of the hottest diets around, and for a good reason. When lectins build up in your body, it can lead to a wide range of chronic issues including severe weight gain.

Luckily, it is very simple to remove the unwanted lectins from your body. All you have to do is watch what you eat. Easier said then done, it can be a little more difficult than you might expect - foods that have lectins in them are not always marked and some of the biggest offenders are hiding in plain sight. To help you navigate in these tricky waters, the following chapters will discuss everything you need to know in order to get started on the right foot with the lectin-free diet.

First, you will learn all about the basics of the diet, as well as the many cons(and a few pros) regarding lectins. Next, you will learn about making the transition to the lectin-free diet, which should only take a few days as long as you do it properly. From there, you will find a host of recipes broken down by category to help ensure that, regardless of what your favorites are, you will be able to find something to enjoy within these pages.

Chapter 1: All About the Lectin-Free Diet

Lectins are a type of protein found in plants, and occasionally in animal protein, that contains a number of negative effects on the body. Some of the biggest lectin offenders are foods like legumes, beans, tomatoes and whole grains. Lectins are a type of protein that helps cells interact with one another more easily when present in the body in small amounts. Plants produce it as a means of keeping insects away and also to help them consume the nitrogen they need in order to grow properly.

This is a problem because when lectins build up in the body they can negatively impact it in a wide variety of ways including things like an increased risk of chronic disease or chronic indigestion. They are categorized as an antinutrient because they block the absorption of many nutrients. If you have ever had a stomachache after eating uncooked beans or other plant foods, then this is likely the reason why. In fact, according to the FDA, consuming just four kidney beans can be enough to cause a wide variety of symptoms including diarrhea, vomiting and nausea.

Good ways to decrease the amount of lectin in your foods include
- Boiling the food
- Fermentation
- Sprouting
- Peeling
- Deseeding
- pressure cooking

Slow cookers typically do not reach a hot enough temperature to remove lectins from the equation and thus, while they are a delicious and effective way to cook a meal, they are not the right choice for these purposes.

While lectins can cause a wide variety of negative effects when they are consumed to excess, they are not all bad. In fact, studies show that small amounts of lectins can actually help good bacteria live in the human digestive tract and do their jobs more effectively. Research has also shown that it can be useful when it comes to diagnosing and identifying various types of cancer. To that end, researchers are even looking at lectin as a potential way to slow down the rate at which cancer cells multiply.

Lectin-free diet

The lectin-free diet was popularized by Dr. Steven Gundry, a former heart surgeon who has since switched his focus to supplement and food-based medicine. According to Gundry, removing lectins from your diet via a lectin-free alternative helps to reduce body weight while improving overall health in the process. It is important to note that the official version of the diet also requires that users purchase a proprietary supplement from Dr. Gundry so following the diet outlined in this book may not be as effective without it. With that being said, this book is **not** recommending going out and purchasing the supplement without doing your own research on its efficacy beforehand.

With that out of the way, the lectin-free diet is all about limiting the amount of lectin in the body to reasonable levels as a means of preventing inflammation from developing due to prolonged exposure. Chronic inflammation is known to lead to everything from arthritis, to cancer, to even death.

Inflammation is not all bad. When it occurs naturally in the body, it can help the body defend against possible infection as well as heal cuts and wounds. If it continues for a prolonged period of time, however, it can lead to a host of illnesses and other negative effects (described in detail in chapter 2), some of which can cause serious long-term consequences when left unchecked. Luckily, there are numerous easy ways to reduce your levels of overall inflammation including changing your eating habits which is where the anti-inflammatory diet comes into play.

As a part of the inflammation process, the body creates an increased amount of immune cells, white blood cells and a substance known as cytokine, as a way to combat infection. There are two primary types of inflammation, the first is a short-term variety that presents itself as swelling, heat, some pain and redness. This is the early phase of inflammation and the symptoms that it brings along with it are caused by the fact that additional blood is flowing to the affected areas in an effort to treat the issue as quickly as possible. This ensures that the troubled spot is protected from additional injury as the body works to fend off irritants, damaged cells, pathogens, viruses and bacteria. Without the inflammation process, even minor cuts and wounds would never heal properly.

On the other hand, chronic inflammation happens slowly over a period of months or years while outwardly presenting no noticeable signs of the ever-growing internal issue. This, in turn, creates a gradual shift in the types of cells that exist around the inflamed spot, as the troubled area will be constantly in a process of destruction and rebirth, sapping bodily resources and slowly festering and becoming something much worse than whatever the initial issue may have been.

Risks of the lectin diet: The lectin-free diet is an especially restrictive diet plan which may naturally make it off limits to some people including children and women who are pregnant and nursing. Those who follow the lectin-free diet also often need to look into alternative types of nutrients, as the lectin-free diet removes a variety of nutritious foods from the rotation as well. It can also be a difficult diet for vegans or vegetarians to follow as whole grains, seeds, nuts and legumes are all, more or less, off limits. As these items also provide much of the body's daily fiber, following the lectin-free diet in the long-term may also cause constipation if alternate types of fiber aren't substituted into the mix.

Foods to eat
- extra virgin olive oil
- olives
- avocado
- mushrooms
- celery
- garlic and onion
- asparagus
- cruciferous vegetables, such as broccoli and Brussels sprouts
- leafy, green vegetables
- cooked sweet potatoes
- A2 milk
- pasture-raised meats

Cooked tubers: Taro root, yucca and sweet potatoes are all excellent sources of vitamins and minerals due to the fact that their roots have strong absorption abilities, drawing minerals from their surroundings. They are also going to be some of your primary sources for fiber as many other common options are off the table.

Leafy greens: Sea vegetables, seaweed, fennel, parsley, endive, spinach, mesclun, kohlrabi and lettuce of all types are all chock full of nutrients and should be a staple of your diet moving forward.

Cruciferous vegetables: Brussel sprouts, cauliflower and broccoli are all great choices when it comes to vegetables that are lectin-free. Onions, mushrooms, celery, garlic and asparagus are all good choices as well. What's more, they are also full of polyphenols.

Avocado: While the avocado is a fruit, it is largely sugar-free and is full of healthy fats and soluble fiber as well. It is a great dietary addition if you are looking to remove antioxidants from your body while losing weight.

Olives and extra virgin olive oil: Olives, and thus olive oil, are full of vitamins and nutrients that are essential if you want to remain healthy while on the lectin-free diet. They are both a great source of potassium, sodium, iron, calcium, vitamin E, vitamin K, fatty acids and polyphenols. They are also known to directly combat inflammatory activities in those who are dealing with autoimmune disorders.

Foods to avoid

- A1 milk
- meat from corn-fed animals
- corn
- If grains are consumed, the plan recommends products made from white flour instead of wheat.
- grains
- fruit, although in-season fruit is allowed in moderation
- potatoes
- nightshade vegetables
- squash
- peanuts
- lentils
- peas
- beans
- eggplants
- tomatoes
- peppers

Legumes and beans: Beans are known to contain more lectins than any other food which means you need to do your absolute best to avoid lentils, peas, beans and any other legume and if you have to eat them, cook them in a pressure cooker first. Additionally, it is important to keep in mind that many legumes hide as nuts which means it is best to remove cashews and peanuts from your diet as well.

Grains: While much of the Standard American Diet is based on grains, the fact of the matter is that humanity as a species has only been eating grains for a relatively limited amount of time which means that, by and large, our bodies haven't caught up yet. As such, eating grain to excess can lead to a host of health problems as your body simply doesn't know what to do with it all. What's more, most grains contain high quantities of lectins which means that if you are going to eat flour you should go with white flour instead as it is devoid of practically everything, including lectin.

Squash: When it comes to remembering what fruits and vegetables to avoid it is important to remember that any vegetable that contains seeds is actually considered a fruit including zucchini, pumpkins and squash. The seeds, as well as the peels, of each of these, are full of lectins which means that if you must eat these things it is vital that you remove the peel and the seeds first.

Nightshades: Nightshade is the classification given to vegetables like eggplant, tomatoes, potatoes and peppers. The peels and seeds of these plants are all high in lectin which means that if you are going to eat them you make sure to deseed, peel and pressure cook them first. Fermentation is also known to reduce the amount of lectin a plant contains.

Corn: Corn is used to fatten up cattle and it has the same effects on humans, largely because it is full of lectins. To eliminate this issue, eliminate all corn, corn syrup and corn-fed meat from your diet, you are sure to start noticing a difference almost immediately.

Casein A1 Milk: While it may sound like a science fiction movie, the fact of the matter is that all the cows in Northern Europe started showing up with a specific genetic mutation a few thousand years ago. While likely caused as a reaction to some long-gone disease, the mutation also added a protein called casein A1 to their milk, which contains a lot of lectins.

Unfortunately, most dairy products are made from milk from casein A1 cows, even if the milk is organic. The only way to avoid getting lectin in this fashion is to either stop consuming most dairy or to specifically purchase milk that has been obtained from unmutated cows, which are designated as Casein A2. Those who believe they are lactose intolerant are likely just reacting to the Casein A1 in their systems.

Ways to further reduce the lectin in your food
While sticking to foods that are low in lectin or are entirely lectin-free is a good goal to keep in mind, sometimes that simply won't be a possibility. When this is the case use the following tips to keep your lectin intake under control as much as possible.

Pressure cook trouble items: If you find yourself on a path to consuming quinoa, regular potatoes, tomatoes or beans, then pressure cooking them first will serve to get rid of a majority of the lectin these foods contain. This doesn't mean you can put anything into it and remove a lectin-free version, however, as the cooker won't be able to do anything about more stubborn foodstuffs like spelt, barley, rye, oats or wheat.

Remove seeds and peels: As a general rule, when following the lectin-free diet you are going to want to deseed and peel anything that can be deseeded or peeled. The part of the fruit or vegetable that contains the greatest concentration of lectin is always going to be the seeds followed by the rind, peel or hull.

White grains only: While you are going to want to avoid grains as much as possible if you do need to consume them always choose the white variety over the brown. While the public perception is that things like white rice and white bread are automatically unhealthy, the fact of the matter is that there are high-quality versions of these items that are just as healthy as the lectin fueled alternatives.

Saving money while eating lectin-free
Much like any special diet, those who follow the lectin-free
diet should expect to pay a little more for groceries than
would otherwise be the case. With this being said, there are
still plenty of things you can do in order to ensure that eating
lectin-free isn't going to break the bank. The goal is not to
focus so much on what you spend and instead pay more
attention to when and how you spend which involves making
three separate shopping lists.

Weekly list: Your weekly shopping list, perhaps
unsurprisingly, is the list that you will be using most often. It
should contain all of the items that you consume most
frequently as well as all the things you need to make specific
meals throughout the week. This is the only list that most
people create which is why their bills are traditionally higher
week to week. As you put together your extended shopping
lists you will find that you will be able to cross more and
more things off your weekly list as a result.

Monthly list: This is the list that you will want to make at the
start of each month and it should mainly stick to the
nonperishable or longer-term items that you may be running
out of. These are the types of things that you will want to buy
in bulk either through wholesale clubs or online retailers.
Once you have a good idea of what types of items will always
be showing up on this list you can then constantly keep an
eye out for deals on them and stock up on the cheap. Great
choices for this list include things like:

- almond flour
- French or Italian butter
- dried herbs/seasonings
- nuts
- unsweetened coconut milk
- stevia
- vinegar

- hot sauce
- frozen vegetables
- olive oil

Seasonal shopping list: This is a list you will only need to make a handful of times per year as it will involve seasonal items that you can stock up on at the beginning of the season and freeze for use for the next few months. This is also when you should shop for free-range fish and pasture-raised meat as buying in bulk here will say you hundreds over a three or four-month period.

Chapter 2: Making the Transition

Once you have decided to make the transition to a lectin-free diet a try, there are going to be a few things you will want to do before taking the plunge, starting with a three-day detox plan design to purge the excess lectin from your system once and for all.

Prepare your body: As your body has adjusted to the amount of lectin that is currently in your system, preparing it to exist in a low-lectin state will require a bit of work. One common den of lectins is processed sugar which has likely led to an increase in bad bacteria in your gut that thrives on it. If you have ever felt a craving for processed sugar or other bad foods then this is likely the reason why. Unfortunately, these cravings and the related mindset they have no doubt created over the years will only make it harder for you to start today.

Nevertheless, you must push them to the side and persevere if you want to start seeing serious changes sooner rather than later. Specifically, it only takes three days to start and you will then begin seeing a marked reduction in inflammation, a more balanced assembly of gut bacteria, weight loss and an improved sense of wellbeing.

Three Day Detox
This three-day detox will help you to remove the majority of the bad bacteria from your gut, making it easier for you to take full advantage of all the recipes in the following chapters by ensuring the transition is as quick and effective as possible. It is important to keep in mind that if you revert back to your old habits then the bad bacteria will return and you will have to go through the whole process from scratch once more.

This is not to say that you can't slip and eat something you know you shouldn't, after all, nobody's perfect, you will only really be in danger if you eat enough of the types of food you should avoid that the negative bacteria will once again feel right at home. While you can certainly skip the three-day cleanse and jump right into the diet proper, taking the time to purge your gut first will ensure you move forward with every possible advantage.

Getting started with the cleanse is simple, all you need to do to start is to say no to certain foods that are high in lectin. Specifically:

- Farm animal proteins
- Inflammatory oils
- Canola
- Soy
- Corn
- Tubers
- Roots
- Nightshade plants
- Soy
- Eggs
- Seeds
- Sugar
- Fruit
- Grains or pseudo-grains
- Dairy

At the same time, you are going to want to ensure that you have plenty of the following vegetables around. You are free to eat as many of them as you like. You can eat them cooked or raw, though if you are already dealing with gut issues or IBS then you will want to ensure you cook them first. Fresh or frozen vegetables are both acceptable as long as they are always organic.

- Mushrooms
- Sea vegetables
- Seaweed

- Algae
- Perilla
- Purslane
- Mint
- Basil
- Parsley
- Mizuna
- Mustard greens
- Escarole
- Fennel
- Butter lettuce
- Dandelion greens
- Endive
- Spinach
- Mesclun
- Kohlrabi
- Romaine
- Leafy greens
- Garlic
- Asparagus
- Okra
- Cilantro
- Hearts of palm
- Artichokes
- Daikon radishes
- Radishes
- Beets
- Artichokes
- Carrot greens
- Carrots
- Chicory
- Scallions
- Chives
- Leeks
- Onions
- Celery

- Nopales cactus
- Kimchi
- Raw sauerkraut
- Radicchio
- Cabbage
- Kale
- Collards
- Watercress
- Arugula
- Swiss chard
- Chinese cabbage
- Napa cabbage
- Bok choy
- Cauliflower
- Brussels sprouts
- Broccoli

Protein: While in the midst of the starter cleanse you will want to limit yourself to small amounts of pastured chicken or wild fish. You will want to split your protein into two, four oz. servings and consume one in the morning and one in the evening to ensure your body continually has everything it needs to run at maximum efficiency.

Fats and oils: During your cleanse you are going to want to try and consume an entire avocado each day. In addition, if you need to cook with oil stick to the following choices that contain low amounts of lectin:

- Flaxseed oil
- Hemp seed oil
- Extra-virgin olive oil
- Walnut oil
- Sesame seed oil
- Macadamia nut oil
- Coconut oil
- Avocado oil

Chapter 3: Breakfast Recipes

Granola cakes

Total Prep & Cooking Time: 75 minutes
Yields: 12 Servings

What to Use
- Salt (1 pinch)
- Vanilla extract (.5 tsp.)
- Cinnamon (1 tsp.)
- Almond butter (.3 c)
- Coconut nectar (.3 c)
- Chia seeds (2 T)
- Pumpkin seed protein powder (2 T)
- Coconut (.5 c)
- Hemp seeds (.5 c)
- Chopped mix nuts (1 c lectin-free)

What to Do
- Place a silicon muffin tray on a baking sheet and set to one side.
- Chop the nuts so the average size is about that of a popcorn kernel and place them in a mixing bowl. Mix in the chia seeds, protein powder, coconut and hemp seeds and mix well.
- Add the coconut nectar to a frying pan before placing the pan on a burner turned to a low/medium heat and stir constantly until it begins to bubble. Mix in the almond butter and continue mixing until it bubbles again.
- Mix in the salt, vanilla and cinnamon and stir vigorously.
- Add the results into the bowl of nuts and stir well to coat. It is important to complete this step quickly as the nectar will harden if it cools.
- Spilt the results into the muffin cups and fill each firmly.
- Place the muffin tray in the refrigerator for 60 minutes to cool.

Lectin-Free Granola

Total Prep & Cooking Time: 20 minutes
Yields: 10 Servings

What to Use
- Raisins (.25 c)
- Coconut oil (1 T)
- Maple syrup (2 T)
- Sea salt (.25 tsp.)
- Cinnamon (1 tsp.)
- Chia seeds (3 T ground)
- Pumpkin seeds (.25 c)
- Coconut (.25 c shredded)
- Almonds (.75 c slivered)
- Walnuts (1 c)

What to Do
- Ensure your oven is heated to 325 degrees F.
- Line a baking sheet using parchment paper
- Add the coconut oil to a saucepan before placing it on top of a burner turned to a high heat. When it is malleable add it to a mixing bowl.
- In the mixing bowl, combine all of the ingredients, save the raisins, in a bowl and mix well.
- Spread the results on the baking sheet in a single layer and place the baking sheet in the oven for 10 minutes. Mix halfway through to ensure it doesn't burn.
- Remove the baking tray from the oven and allow it to cool before adding in the raisins.

Lectin-free cereal

Total Prep & Cooking Time: 5 minutes
Yields: 1 Serving

What to Use
- Cacao nibs (1 pinch)
- Goji berries (1 small handful)
- Coconut flakes (1 small handful)
- Almonds (1 small handful)
- Walnuts (1 small handful)
- Pecans (1 small handful)

What to Do
- Add all of the ingredients to a cereal bowl and mix well.
- Top with A2 milk.
- Enjoy!

Pumpkin spice pancakes

Total Prep & Cooking Time: 15 minutes
Yields: 6 Servings

What to Use
- Coconut oil (2 T)
- Coconut sugar (1 T)
- Coconut milk (2 T)
- Apple cider vinegar (.25 tsp.)
- Baking soda (.5 tsp.)
- Eggs (3)
- Vanilla (.25 tsp.)
- Sea salt (.25 tsp.)
- Pumpkin pie spice (1 tsp.)
- Pumpkin puree (.3 c)
- Coconut flour (.25 c)

What to Do
- Add all of the ingredients to a mixing bowl and combine thoroughly using a hand blender. Continue to blend until all of the lumps in the batter have been removed.
- Add the coconut oil to a skillet before placing it on the stove over a burner turned to a medium heat. After the pan has warmed appropriately add in .3 c of the batter and shape it using a spoon. Let each pancake cook about 2 minutes per side.

Apple Pie Pancakes

Total Prep & Cooking Time: 25 minutes
Yields: 18 Servings

What to Use
- Raw honey (4 T divided)
- Coconut oil (3 T)
- A2 milk (3 T)
- Salt (1 pinch)
- Nutmeg (1 pinch)
- Cinnamon (1 tsp.)
- Baking soda (.5 tsp.)
- Coconut flour (.5 c)
- Vanilla extract (1 tsp.)
- A2 Milk (1 c)
- Eggs (4)
- Cinnamon (2 tsp.)
- Apples (2 c diced)
- Coconut oil (1 T)

What to Do
- Add the coconut oil to a skillet before placing it on top of a burner turned to a medium heat and let it warm before adding in the cinnamon and apples. Allow them to cook about 8 minutes.
- At the same time, add the vanilla, honey, milk and eggs to a mixing bowl and combining thoroughly before adding in the salt, nutmeg, cinnamon, baking soda and coconut flour.
- After the apples have finished cooking, add in half of the apples to the batter and mix well.
- Add the remaining coconut oil, raw honey and 3 T milk to the skillet and stir while the oil melts. Remove from the burner and set aside.
- Add the coconut oil to a skillet before placing it on the stove over a burner turned to a medium heat. After the pan has warmed appropriately add in .3 c of the

batter and shape it using a spoon. Let each pancake cook about 2 minutes per side.

Sweet potato pancakes

Total Prep & Cooking Time: 20 minutes
Yields: 6 Servings

What to Use
- Coconut oil (2 T)
- Eggs (4)
- Sea salt (1 pinch)
- Nutmeg (.5 tsp.)
- Cinnamon (.5 tsp.)
- Vanilla extract (1 tsp.)
- Nut butter (.5 c)
- Sweet potato (1 chopped, peeled)

What to Do
- Cook the sweet potato in a pressure cooker to remove as much lectin as possible.
- Add the sweet potato to a mixing bowl and mash thoroughly before adding in 4 egg yolks and the nut butter and mix well. Mix in the salt, nutmeg, cinnamon and vanilla.
- In a separate bowl, beat the egg whites until they are stiff enough to stand alone before adding them to the batter. This is important to ensure your pancakes come out as fluffy as possible.
- Add the coconut oil to a skillet before placing it on the stove over a burner turned to a medium heat. After the pan has warmed appropriately add in .3 c of the batter and shape it using a spoon. Let each pancake cook about 2 minutes per side.

Banana Bread

Total Prep & Cooking Time: 65 minutes
Yields: 6 Servings

What to Use
- Cacao nibs (.5 c)
- Raw honey (.5 c)
- Bananas (1 c mashed)
- Eggs (3 room temp)
- Coconut oil (2 T melted)
- Coconut flour (.25 c)
- Almond flour (.75 c)
- Sea salt (.5 tsp.)
- Baking soda (.75 tsp.)

What to Do
- Ensure your oven is heated to 350 degrees F
- Add all of the dry ingredients to a mixing bowl and whisk well.
- Separately, combine all of the wet ingredients and then mix the two bowls together. Use a mixer if needed to ensure batter is blended well.
- Grease a baking pan using coconut oil before adding in the batter and placing the pan in the oven for 45 minutes.
- You will know the bread is ready when you can stick a knife into the center of it and pull it out clean.

Pumpkin Cranberry Muffins

Total Prep & Cooking Time: 45minutes
Yields: 12 Servings

What to Use
- Orange zest (1 orange)
- Cranberries (1 c)
- Vanilla extract (1 tsp.)
- Palm shortening (.25 c)
- Raw honey (.5 c)
- Eggs (4)
- Pumpkin puree (1 c)
- Cloves (1 tsp.)
- Cinnamon (1 T)
- Sea salt (.5 tsp.)
- Baking powder (.5 tsp.)
- Baking soda (.5 tsp.)
- Coconut flour (.5 c)
- Tapioca flour (.3 c)

What to Do
- Ensure your oven is heated to 350 degrees F
- Fill a standard muffin tin with paper liners
- Add the spices, salt, baking powder, baking soda, coconut flour and tapioca flour to a mixing bowl and combine thoroughly.
- In a separate bowl, mix together the vanilla, shortening, honey, eggs and pumpkin and mix until it is completely smooth.
- Combine the two bowls and mix until smooth before adding in the zest and the cranberries.
- Add the batter to the muffin tin before placing the tin in the oven for 25 minutes. You will know the muffins are ready when you can stick a toothpick into the center muffin and pull it out clean.

Fruit Souffle

Total Prep & Cooking Time: 35 minutes
Yields: 2 Servings

What to Use
- Coconut oil (1 T)
- Mixed frozen fruit (1 c)
- Cinnamon (2 tsp.)
- Vanilla (2 tsp.)
- Raw honey (2 T)
- Eggs (4 room temp, whites and yolks separated)

What to Do
- Ensure your oven is heated to 350 degrees F,
- Add the fruit and coconut oil to a pair of large ramekins. Add the ramekins to the oven while it is preheating to melt the oil and soften the fruit.
- Add the egg whites to a stand mixer and whisk until they begin to solidify.
- In a separate bowl, mix together the yolks, cinnamon, vanilla and raw honey.
- Combine the two egg mixtures and whisk briefly until they incorporate. Shoot for 5 seconds, do not over mix.
- Remove the ramekins from the oven and slice the fruit before adding in the egg mixture to each.
- Place the ramekins back in the oven for about 16 minutes.

Lectin-Free Hash

Total Prep & Cooking Time: 35 minutes
Yields: 3 Servings

What to Use
- Sage (1 T minced)
- Sweet potato (1 large, cubed)
- Coconut oil (2 T)
- Cinnamon (1 tsp.)
- Apple (1 cubed)
- Onion (1 chopped fine)
- Pancetta (6 oz. diced)

What to Do
- Add the pancetta to a skillet before placing it on top of a burner turned to a low/medium heat. Allow it to cook about 3 minutes before removing it from the skillet while retaining the fat.
- Add the cinnamon, apples and onion to the skillet and allow everything to cook about 7 minutes.
- Remove the ingredients from the pan and add them to the pancetta.
- Ensure there is still fat in the skillet before adding in the potatoes and letting them cook about 2 minutes before stirring well and then cooking another 2 minutes. Continue cooking and stirring until the potatoes have browned completely.
- Add everything back to the pan and mix in the sage. Let everything warm prior to serving.

Yummy Pork Recipe

Total Prep & Cooking Time: 25 minutes
Yields: 6 patties

What to Use
- Red pepper flakes (.5 tsp.)
- Raw honey (2 tsp.)
- Oregano (1 tsp. dried)
- Basil 91 tsp. dried)
- Black pepper (1 tsp.)
- Chili powder (1 tsp.)
- Thyme (.5 tsp.)
- Sage (1 tsp. ground)
- Sea salt (2 tsp.)
- Parsley (2 tsp. minced)
- Onion (.3 c pureed)
- Turkey (1.25 lbs. ground)
- Pork (2 lbs. ground)

What to Do
- Add all the seasonings to a mixing and mix well before adding in the onion, syrup and meat. Use your hands to combine thoroughly and then shape into 6 patties.
- Add the coconut oil to a skillet before placing it on the stove over a burner turned to a medium/high heat. Cook each patty about 2 minutes per side.

Breakfast skillet

Total Prep & Cooking Time: 25 minutes
Yields: 4 Servings

What to Use
- Water (.5 c)
- Onion powder (.5 tsp.)
- Pepper (.5 tsp.)
- Salt (.5 tsp.)
- Homemade breakfast sausage (1 lb.)
- Coconut oil (1 T)
- Butternut squash (12 oz. cubed)

What to Do
- Add 1 T coconut oil to the skillet before placing it on the stove over a burner turned to a high/medium heat.
- Add the butternut squash to the pan and allow it to sauté for about 2 minutes.
- Add in the water, before letting everything cook, for about 4 minutes or until the water has been completely absorbed.
- Move the squash to the sides of the pan before adding the sausage to allow it to brown. Do not mix the two until the sausage has completely browned.
- Mix all of the ingredients together and season as desired before cooking an additional 60 seconds.
- Serve hot.

Eggs and sweet potato hash browns

Total Prep & Cooking Time: 20 minutes
Yields: 2 Servings

What to Use
- Eggs (4)
- Sweet potato (1 peeled, skinned)

What to Do
- Ensure your oven is heated to 400 degrees F.
- Prepare a muffin tin by greasing it using coconut oil.
- Grate the sweet potato using a cheese grater and collect the shavings in a mixing bowl. Fill the muffin tin with the sweet potato shavings and press down well to create a crust.
- Place the muffin tin in the oven for 5 minutes, take care not to burn the sweet potato.
- Remove the tin from the oven and crack an egg into each section of sweet potato crust. Return the muffin tin back to the oven and let everything bake an additional 10 minutes.
- Let cool prior to removing from tin and serving.

Shepherd pie

Total Prep & Cooking Time: 35 minutes
Yields: 4 Servings

What to Use
- Hot sauce (3 T)
- Avocado (.5 sliced)
- Cheddar Jack cheese (.3 c)
- Bacon (6 slices cooked)
- Pepper (.25 tsp.)
- Cumin (.25 tsp.)
- Chili powder (.25 tsp.)
- Paprika (.25 tsp.)
- Sea salt (.5 tsp.)
- Egg (1 beaten)
- Coconut flour (2 T)
- Cauliflower (.5 c grated)
- A2 milk (2 T)
- Eggs (4 beaten)

What to Do
- Ensure your oven is heated to 400 degrees F.
- Prepare 4 ramekins for use by greasing them with coconut oil.
- Add the salt, pepper, milk and eggs to a large mixing bowl and combine thoroughly. Add the results evenly to the ramekins and place them in the oven for 10 minutes.
- Remove the ramekins from the oven and allow them to cool before layering 2 bacon slices on top of each.
- In a large mixing bowl combine the pepper, cumin, chili powder, paprika, salt, cheese, egg, coconut flour, and cauliflower and mix well. Split the results into the ramekins and spread evenly.
- Brush the tops of the ramekins using coconut oil before placing them back in the oven for 20 minutes.

- Let cool prior to serving.

Kale Scramble

Total Prep & Cooking Time: 10 minutes
Yields: 1 Serving

What to Use
- Pepper (as desired)
- Salt (as desired)
- Coconut oil (1 T)
- Garlic powder (1 tsp.)
- Turmeric (1.5 tsp.)
- Kale (1 c chopped)
- Eggs (2)

What to Do
- Add the coconut oil to a skillet before placing it on the stove over a burner turned to a medium heat.
- Whisk the eggs in a small bowl and set aside.
- Add the kale to the skillet and allow it to wilt slightly before adding in the eggs, pepper, salt, garlic powder and turmeric.
- Let everything cook until the eggs reach your desired consistency.

Lectin-free burrito

Total Prep & Cooking Time: 15 minutes
Yields: 4 Servings

What to Use
  • Black pepper (as desired)
  • Sea salt (as desired)
  • Gluten-free flour tortillas (4)
  • Onion (.5 diced)
  • Cheddar cheese (.75 c died)
  • Eggs (4)
  • Coconut oil (2 T)

What to Do
  • Add the coconut oil to a skillet before placing it on the stove over a burner turned to a medium heat. Add in the onions and allow them to cook for about 3 minutes until they begin to brown.
  • Add in the salt, eggs and cheese and scramble the eggs until they reach your desired consistency and remove from skillet.
  • Warm tortillas in oven.
  • Split ingredients in fourths between tortillas prior to serving.

Cheese and Artichoke Quiche

Total Prep & Cooking Time: 35 minutes
Yields: 6 Servings

What to Use
- Black pepper (as desired)
- Sea salt (.25 tsp.)
- Nutmeg (1 dash)
- Rosemary leaves (.5 tsp. ground)
- Cheddar cheese (2 c shredded)
- Eggs (5 beaten)
- Artichoke hearts (1 c chopped)
- Garlic (2 cloves minced)
- Red onion (1 sliced)

What to Do
- Ensure your oven is heated to 350 degrees F.
- Prepare a quiche pan by greasing it with coconut oil.
- Add all of the ingredients to a mixing bowl and combine thoroughly.
- Pour the results into the quiche pan and ensure it is even.
- Place the quiche pan in the oven and let it cook approximately 25 minutes. You will know it is ready when you can push a toothpick through the center and pull it out clean.
- Let cool 5 minutes prior to serving.

Pumpkin bagels

Total Prep & Cooking Time: 35 minutes
Yields: 8 Servings

What to Use
- Apple cider vinegar (1 tsp.)
- Baking soda (.5 tsp.)
- Raw honey (1.5 T)
- Sea salt (1 pinch)
- Cinnamon (.5 tsp.)
- Pumpkin pie spice (1.25 tsp.)
- Vanilla extract (1 tsp.)
- Pumpkin puree (.5 c)
- Coconut oil (2 T)
- Eggs (3 beaten)
- Golden flax meal (3 T)

What to Do
- Ensure your oven is heated to 350 degrees F.
- Prepare a bagel pan by greasing it with coconut oil.
- Add the sea salt, cinnamon, pumpkin pie spice, golden flax meal and coconut flour to a large mixing bowl and mix well.
- Separately, mix together honey, vanilla extract, milk of choice, pumpkin puree, coconut oil and egg.
- Combine the vinegar and baking soda together and mix well before quickly adding the fizzing results to the egg mixture.
- Combine the two bowl and mix until smooth.
- Add the batter to the pan and ensure the space for the hole is clean.
- Place the pan in the oven for about 25 minutes or until the tops are browned and firm.
- Allow bagels to cool completely prior to removing them from the pan.

Coconut banana muffins

Total Prep & Cooking Time: 20 minutes
Yields: 40 mini muffins

What to Use
- Cinnamon (1 tsp.)
- Coconut oil (.5 c)
- Vanilla extract (1 tsp.)
- Bananas (4 mashed)
- Coconut (.25 c shredded)
- Coconut sugar (.25 c)
- Eggs (2)
- Sea salt (1 tsp.)
- Baking soda (1 tsp.)
- All-purpose flour (2 c)

What to Do
- Ensure your oven is heated to 350 degrees F.
- Add liners to two mini muffin pans.
- Add all of the dry ingredients to a large mixing bowl and combine thoroughly. Retain 1 T shredded coconut.
- Beat the eggs in a separate bowl before adding them to the dry ingredients bowl and mix well. Add in the rest of the wet ingredients and mix until the batter is sticky but do not overmix.
- Add the batter to the mini muffin pans before placing them in the oven for about 15 minutes.
- Top with remaining coconut prior to serving.

Apple bread

Total Prep & Cooking Time: 80 minutes
Yields: 4 Servings

What to Use
- Organic cinnamon (1 tsp.)
- Coconut oil (.5 c)
- Water (.3 c filtered)
- Apple cider vinegar (1 T)
- Vanilla extract (1 tsp.)
- Apple (2 c diced)
- Coconut sugar (.25 c)
- Eggs (2)
- Sea salt (1 tsp.)
- Baking powder (1 tsp.)
- Baking soda (1 tsp.)
- All-purpose flour (2 c)

What to Do
- Ensure your oven is heated to 350 degrees F.
- Prepare a loaf pan by greasing it with coconut oil.
- Add all of the dry ingredients to a large mixing bowl and combine thoroughly.
- Beat the eggs in a separate bowl before adding them to the dry ingredients bowl and mix well. Add in the rest of the wet ingredients and mix until the batter is sticky but do not overmix.
- Add the batter to the pan before placing it in the oven and letting it cook about 65 minutes.

Spinach Frittata

Total Prep & Cooking Time: 40 minutes
Yields: 4 Servings

What to Use
- Salt (as desired)
- Pepper (as desired)
- Coconut oil (2 T)
- Cheese (5.3 oz. shredded)
- Bacon (5.3 oz.)
- Spinach (8 oz.)
- Heavy whipping cream (1 c)
- Eggs (8)

What to Do
- Start by making sure your oven is heated to 350F.
- Add the oil to a pan before placing the pan on the stove over a burner turned to a high/medium heat and let it melt before adding in the bacon and allowing it to fry until crispy before adding in the spinach.
- In a small mixing bowl, combine the heavy whipping cream and eggs and whisk well.
- Add the results to a prepared baking dish before crumbling the bacon and adding it, the cheese and the egg to the mixture and combining thoroughly.
- Place the dish in the oven and let it bake for approximately 25 minutes.
- Let cool 5 minutes prior to serving.

Chapter 4: Lunch Recipes

Celery soup

Total Prep & Cooking Time: 30 minutes
Yields: 4 Servings

What to Use
- Black pepper (as desired)
- Sea salt (as desired)
- Coconut milk (1 c)
- Yellow onion (1 chopped)
- Water (2 c)
- Dill (.5 tsp.)
- Sea salt (1 pinch)
- Celery (1 bunch chopped)

What to Do
- Add all of the ingredients to an Instant Pot and mix well. Seal the lid and choose the option for soup. This will warm the soup for 30 minutes before switching to a warming mode for a few hours.
- Once the timer goes off select the option to manually vent the pressure.
- Add the ingredients to an immersion blender and blend well.
- Serve hot.

Sausage Risotto

Total Prep & Cooking Time: 30 minutes
Yields: 4 Servings

What to Use
- Coconut oil (1 T)
- Summer squash (2 diced, seeded)
- Onions (2 c sliced)
- Cajun seasoning (1 T)
- Water (3.5 c)
- Leafy greens (2 handfuls chopped)
- Rope sausage (1.5 lbs. diagonally sliced)
- Arborio rice (2 c)
- Bell peppers (1.5 c diced)

What to Do
- Add the spices and the salt to a small bowl and mix well before sprinkling over the top of the sausage and rubbing well.
- Turn your pressure cooker to a high/medium heat and add in the coconut oil and allow it to melt before adding in the sausage and allowing it to cook about 3 minutes.
- Add in the remaining ingredients and stir well before cooking an additional 3 minutes.
- Sir in the remaining ingredients and close the lid before selecting the option for high heat and full pressure. Let everything cook for 5 minutes before letting it sit for 5 minutes and letting the pressure release an addition 3 minutes.
- Add in the remaining seasoning and stir well prior to serving.

Chicken and Celery Fries

Total Prep & Cooking Time: 35 minutes
Yields: 6 Servings

What to Use-Chicken
- Olive oil (2 T)
- Black pepper (.25 tsp.)
- Salt (.5 tsp.)
- Chicken breasts (4)

What to Use-fries
- Black pepper (.25 tsp.)
- Salt (.5 tsp.)
- Olive oil (2 T)
- Celery (1.5 lbs.)

What to Do
- Start by making sure your oven is heated to 400 degrees F.
- Cut chicken into small pieces and place into a large mixing bowl before coating in oil and seasoning using spices. Let it marinate for a minimum of 15 minutes.
- While the chicken marinates, cut the celery into strips before adding to a separate mixing bowl, coating in oil and seasoning with salt and pepper. Shake well.
- Add the fries to a baking sheet and place them in the oven to bake 20 minutes.
- Broil the chicken until its internal temperature reads at least 165 degrees Fahrenheit.

Sloppy Joe

Total Prep & Cooking Time: 75 minutes
Yields: 6 Servings

What to Use
- Black pepper (as desired)
- Sea salt (as desired)
- Avocado oil (1 T)
- Pistachios (.25 c shelled)
- Water (.75 c)
- Chili (1 crushed)
- Paprika (.5 tsp.)
- Ginger (1 T minced)
- Garam masala (1 tsp.)
- Avocado oil (2 T)
- Garlic (1 clove minced)
- Avocado (1 mashed)
- Ground turkey (1 lb.)
- Avocado oil (2 T)
- White onion (.3 c diced fine)
- Cumin (1 tsp.)
- Apple cider vinegar (1 tsp.)
- Coconut milk (.25 c)
- Cilantro (1 handful chopped)

What to Do
- Add 2 T avocado oil to a skillet before placing it on the stove over a burner turned to a medium/low heat and add in the pistachios. Allow them to cook about 4 minutes and set aside.
- Add 2 T avocado oil to a pot before placing in on a burner turned to a medium heat and adding in the ginger and garlic. Allow them to brown for 60 seconds before adding in the garam masala, water, mashed avocado, salt, paprika and chili. Allow the pot to simmer, covered while you complete the next steps.

- Add the remaining avocado oil to the skillet before adding in the cumin and onions and stirring for 5 minutes before adding in the beef and the chilis. Brown the meat completely.
- Add the skillet ingredients to the pot and turn up the heat to allow it to boil, removing the lid slightly to vent. Simmer for an additional 15 minutes on low/medium heat.
- Add in the pistachios, vinegar and coconut milk and mix well prior to serving. Garnish with cilantro.

Ravioli and pesto

Total Prep & Cooking Time: 35 minutes
Yields: 1 Serving

What to Use
- Parmesan cheese (.25 c)
- Mascarpone (.25 c)
- Coconut wraps (5)
- Eggs (2 beaten with 1 tsp. water)
- Coconut oil (4 T + .5 c divided)
- Frozen spinach (10 oz. thawed, dried)
- Pine nuts (.25 c)
- Garlic (2 cloves)
- Parmesan cheese (1 oz.)
- Basil leaves (2 c)
- Balsamic vinegar (as desired)
- Mixed salad greens (5 oz.)

What to Do
- Ensure your oven is heated to 350 degrees F.
- Add the coconut oil to a skillet before placing it on the stove over a burner turned to a medium heat. Add in the spinach and let it cook 2 minutes before removing it and placing it in a mixing bowl.
- Add the .25 c parmesan cheese and the mascarpone to the bowl and mix well to combine thoroughly.
- Line up 50 percent of the wraps on a cutting board before brushing them using the water and egg mixture. Place 1 T of the spinach mixture into each corner of each wrap, leaving as much space as possible between the scoops.
- Brush one of the remaining wraps with the egg mixture and then use it to cover the tops of the filled wraps. Press down on the edges to create pockets and then use a ravioli cutter to cut out four squares total.
- Add the remaining ingredients to a blender and blend well to create the pesto.

- Place the rest of the coconut oil into a pan before placing the pan on the stove over a burner turned to a medium heat. Add the ravioli to the pan in batches, each should take about 2 minutes to cook, flip them at the 1-minute mark.

Enchiladas

Total Prep & Cooking Time: 45 minutes
Yields: 8 Servings

What to Use
- Black pepper (as desired)
- Sea salt (as desired)
- Raw honey (1 tsp.)
- Paprika (.25 tsp.)
- Coconut aminos (1 tsp.)
- Oregano (.5 tsp. dried)
- Flour tortillas (8 warmed)
- Bone broth (2 c divided)
- Chicken (8 oz. shredded)
- Goat cheese (8 oz. crumbled)
- Cumin (.5 tsp. ground)
- Apple cider vinegar (3 tsp.)
- Garlic (4 cloves peeled)
- Shiitake mushrooms (8 oz. chopped)
- Olive oil (2 T)

What to Do
- Ensure your oven is heated to 400 degrees F.
- Add the oil to a skillet before placing it on the stove over a burner turned to a medium/high heat. Add in the mushrooms and onions and allow them to cook about 6 minutes, stirring regularly.
- Mix in the pepper, salt and .5 c broth before reducing the heat to medium and letting everything cook about 4 minutes.
- Once all the broth has been absorbed you will want to place all of the ingredients into a mixing bowl before stirring in half of the goat cheese.
- Add the rest of the broth, paprika, oregano, honey, cumin, 2 tsp. sea salt, coconut aminos, garlic, apple cider vinegar and the rest of the broth in a blender

and pulse until smooth. Add .5 c of the sauce to a glass dish (9 x 13).

- Add .25 c of the mushroom mixture to each tortilla before folding up the bottom and then rolling it tightly. Place the finished tortillas into the baking dish and cover them with the sauce. Top all of the tortillas with the rest of the sauce and the remaining cheese.
- Place the baking dish in the oven for about 15 minutes. You will know they are ready when the cheese is melted and the sauce is bubbling.

Baked sweet potato

Total Prep & Cooking Time: 20 minutes
Yields: 2 Servings

What to Use
- Black pepper (as desired)
- Sea salt (as desired)
- Garlic (.25 tsp.)
- Kale (.5 c)
- Olive oil (.25 tsp.)
- Sweet potato (6 oz.)

What to Do
- Ensure your oven is heated to 350 degrees F.
- Add the sweet potatoes to pieces of aluminum foil, taking care to pierce the potato in numerous places to allow for venting. Coat the potatoes in the foil and then place them on a baking sheet.
- Place the baking sheet in the oven and let them cook for 30 minutes, you will know they are ready when they are soft all the way through.
- Once they are finished cooking, remove the potatoes from the foil and place them in a large bowl. Mash the potatoes with the salt, pepper, garlic, olive oil and kale.

Bok choy and fried shrimp

Total Prep & Cooking Time: 10 minutes
Yields: 4 Servings

What to Use
- Bok choy (.75 c)
- Garlic (.5 tsp.)
- Ginger (.25 tsp.)
- Sesame oil (.25 tsp.)
- Wild shrimp (24 oz.)

What to Do
- Add all of the ingredients to a wok and stir-fry for 10 minutes.
- Serve hot.

Fettuccine

Total Prep & Cooking Time: 30 minutes
Yields: 4 Servings

What to Use
- Black pepper (as desired)
- Sea salt (as desired)
- Mascarpone (1 c)
- Asparagus (1 bunch chopped)
- Parmesan cheese (.25 c grated)
- Shitake mushrooms (5 oz. sliced)
- Shirataki fettuccine noodles (32 oz. cooked)
- Extra-virgin olive oil (.25 c)
- Italian parsley (.5 c)
- Italian seasoning (.5 tsp.)

What to Do
- Cook the pasta according to the provided instructions and keep 1 c of the water used to cook the noodles.
- Add the oil to a skillet before placing it on the stove over a burner turned to a medium heat. Add in the mushrooms and increase the heat to high/medium and cook for 2 minutes before adding in the asparagus, the remaining oil and .5 tsp. salt. Cook until the asparagus is tender and crisp which should be about 3 minutes.
- Turn off the heat before adding in the mascarpone and shirataki noodles before tossing to coat. Add .25 c of the reserved noodle water at a time to thin the sauce and keep the noodles moist. Stir in the remaining ingredients and serve warm.

Meatballs and Salad

Total Prep & Cooking Time: 45 minutes
Yields: 6 Servings

What to Use
- Black pepper (as desired)
- Sea salt (as desired)
- Raw honey (2 tsp.)
- Coconut aminos (1 T)
- Sesame coconut oil (1 T)
- Red pepper (.5 tsp.)
- Lime juice (3 T)
- Scallions (4 sliced thin)
- Cilantro (.5 c)
- Shitake mushrooms (.5 c sautéed)
- Meatballs (12 cooked)
- Baby bok choy (6 heads)
- Coconut oil (2 T)

What to Do
- Add the coconut oil to a skillet before placing it on the stove over a burner turned to a medium heat. Add in the mushrooms and allow them to cook for about 5 minutes. Add in the meatballs and let everything cook until they are warm.
- In a serving bowl, add the honey, coconut aminos, sesame oil, red pepper and lime juice and mix well. Add in the scallions, cilantro, bok choy and the mixture from the skillet and toss to coat.

Coconut chicken

Total Prep & Cooking Time: 30 minutes
Yields: 4 Servings

What to Use
- Black pepper (as desired)
- Sea salt (as desired)
- Coconut milk (1 c)
- 5 spice powder (1 tsp.)
- Kosher salt (1 tsp.)
- Coconut aminos (3 T)
- Drumsticks (10 skin removed)
- Onion (1 sliced thin, peeled)
- Fish sauce (2 T)
- Ginger (1 in. peeled, chopped)
- Cilantro (.25 c)
- Garlic (4 cloves crushed, peeled)
- Lime juice (1 lime)
- Lemongrass (1 stalk chopped, skinned)
- Coconut oil (1 tsp.)

What to Do
- Add the ginger, fish sauce, garlic, lemongrass, coconut aminos and 5 spice powder in a blender before adding in the coconut milk and using the pulse setting to blend.
- Add the drumsticks to a bowl and season as desired before adding in the blender mixture and ensuring the drumsticks are well-coated.
- Turn on your Instant Pot and set it to the sauté setting and allow it to heat up before adding in the sliced onions and coconut oil and letting them cook about 5 minutes.
- Add the drumsticks and the marinade to the Instant Pot and select the warm option before sealing and locking the lid.

- Select the Manual option and then set the timer for 15 minutes and high pressure.
- Use the manual release valve when the drumsticks are done.
- Season with fish sauce prior to serving.

Arugula salad with sweet potato

Total Prep & Cooking Time: 20 minutes
Yields: 4 Servings

What to Use
- Black pepper (as desired)
- Sea salt (as desired)
- Parmesan cheese (.25 c)
- Baby arugula (5 oz.)
- Dijon mustard (1 T)
- White wine vinegar (1 T)
- Swiss cheese (2 oz. shredded)
- Prosciutto (2 oz.)
- Sweet potato (1 lb. cubed, peeled)
- Coconut oil (.25 c)
- Tarragon leaves (.25 c chopped)

What to Do
- Add your sweet potatoes to a boiler and then cover them with water. Allow them to boil before adding some salt and then reducing the temperature to let them simmer about 12 minutes. After they are done cooking, drain them, run cold water over them and then deposit them on a cutting board and dice them.
- In a small bowl, combine the pepper, mustard, salt, oil and vinegar and mix well.
- Split the arugula between 4 bowls before adding in the tarragon, sweet potatoes, prosciutto and swiss cheese. Top with dressing and parmesan prior to serving.

Chicken and cabbage with apples and cranberries

Total Prep & Cooking Time: 35 minutes
Yields: 4 Servings

What to Use
- Black pepper (as desired)
- Sea salt (as desired)
- Apple cider vinegar (1 T)
- Ginger (1 tsp. ground)
- Chicken bone broth (.5 c)
- Apples (2 sliced)
- Chicken breast (2 lbs. boneless, skinless)
- Cranberries (1 c frozen)
- Raw honey (1 T)
- Cabbage (1 head cored)
- Cinnamon (1 tsp.)

What to Do
- Add all of the ingredients to your Instant Pot and select the poultry setting prior to closing and securing the lid. Set the timer for 20 minutes.
- Allow the pressure to release naturally for 10 minutes.
- Serve hot and enjoy!

Mushroom mini pizza

Total Prep & Cooking Time: 35 minutes
Yields: 2 Servings

What to Use
- Black pepper (as desired)
- Sea salt (as desired)
- Prosciutto (2 slices)
- Buffalo mozzarella (1 ball sliced)
- Basil pesto (6 T)
- Coconut oil (2 T)
- Portobello mushrooms (2 caps)

What to Do
- Ensure your oven is heated to 325 degrees F.
- Add the mushrooms caps to a baking pan before coating them in coconut oil. Place them in the oven for 5 minutes before removing the baking sheet from the oven, flipping the mushroom caps and returning them to the oven for an additional 5 minutes. The end result should be both crispy and brown on top.
- Add 3 T pesto to each cap, top with a slice of prosciutto and then the mozzarella.
- Return the mushrooms to the baking sheet and return the sheet to the oven for an additional 5 minutes.
- Season prior to serving hot.

Orange salmon salad

Total Prep & Cooking Time: 30 minutes
Yields: 4 Servings

What to Use
- Black pepper (as desired)
- Sea salt (as desired)
- Dijon mustard (1 tsp.)
- Coconut oil (4 T)
- White wine vinegar (3 T)
- Raw honey (1 tsp.)
- Dill (1 T chopped)
- Lemon juice (1 lemon)
- Navel oranges (2 sectioned, peeled)
- Red onion (1 sliced thin)
- Salmon (1 lb. broiled, flaked)
- Baby spinach (5 oz.)
- Feta cheese (2 oz. crumbled)
- Hazelnuts (.3 c chopped, toasted)

What to Do
- In a serving bowl, combine the flaked salmon, navel orange pieces, spinach and red onions.
- In a separate bowl, add the feta cheese and hazelnuts and toss to combine before combining the two bowls and mixing well.
- In a small bowl, mix together the Dijon mustard, coconut oil, white wine vinegar, honey, dill and lemon juice and whisk well.
- Add the dressing to the salad and toss to coat.

Chapter 5: Dinner Recipes

Spinach salad with steak

Total Prep & Cooking Time: 25 minutes
Yields: 4 Servings

What to Use
- Black pepper (as desired)
- Sea salt (as desired)
- Red wine vinegar (2 T)
- Thyme (2 tsp. dried)
- Goat milk yogurt (4 oz.)
- Shirataki rice (1 c rinsed, drained)
- Baby spinach (5 oz.)
- Grass-fed steak (1 lb.)
- Pine nuts (2 T)

What to Do
- Add the steak to a skillet before placing it on the stove over a burner turned to a medium heat. Prepare your steak to its desired level of doneness.
- While the steak is cooking, add the pepper, salt, thyme, yogurt and red wine vinegar in a small bowl and whisk well.
- Cook the rice according to instructions.
- Plate the spinach in four separate bowls before topping with sliced steak, pine nuts, rice and dressing.

Noodles with broccoli and pesto

Total Prep & Cooking Time: 20 minutes
Yields: 4 Servings

What to Use
- Black pepper (as desired)
- Sea salt (as desired)
- Broccoli florets (1 c)
- Olive oil (.25 tsp.)
- Basil pesto (.5 c)
- Miracle noodles (1 bag cooked)

What to Do
- Add the coconut oil to a skillet before placing it on the stove over a burner turned to a medium heat. Add in the broccoli florets, pesto and noodles and let everything cook about 10 minutes, mixing regularly.
- Season as desired prior to serving.

Squash soup

Total Prep & Cooking Time: 45 minutes
Yields: 4 Servings

What to Use
- Black pepper (as desired)
- Sea salt (as desired)
- Thyme (2 T)
- Chives (2 T)
- Coconut milk (1 can)
- Oregano (2 T)
- Chicken stock (6 c)
- Garlic (4 cloves peeled)
- Celery (2 c)
- Salt (1.5 T)
- Herbs de Provence 93 T)
- Carrots (3)
- Cayenne pepper (.25 T)
- Onion (1 sliced)
- Butternut squash (1 peeled)
- Parsley leaves (.25 c)

What to Do
- Slice the butternut squash in half before trimming off the ends and removing the seeds. Dice the remaining squash.
- Add all of the ingredients, except the coconut milk to your pressure cooker, saving the chicken stock and seasonings for last.
- Secure the lid of the pressure cooker and choose the soup option. Allow the Instant Pot to cook for 30 minutes and then release the pressure manually.
- Pour the results into an immersion blender and blend your soup until smooth.
- Add in the coconut milk and season as desired.
- Serve hot.

Sweet potato gnocchi

Total Prep & Cooking Time: 60 minutes
Yields: 4 Servings

What to Use
- Black pepper (as desired)
- Sea salt (as desired)
- Parmesan cheese (.25 c)
- Lemon (1 zested, juiced)
- Garlic (1 clove crushed)
- Coconut oil (3 T)
- Basil (.5 c torn, divided)
- Sweet potato (peeled, chunked)
- Egg (1)
- Sea salt (.5 tsp.)
- Cassava flour (.5 c)

What to Do
- Place the sweet potatoes in a pot before filling the pot with water so the gnocchi is covered in about 2 inches of water before placing the pot on the stove over a burner turned to a high heat. Bring the pot to a boil before turning down the heat and allowing the pot to simmer for 15 minutes partially covered. Drain the potatoes, rinse them with cold water, and then drain.
- Place the sweet potatoes in a bowl and mash them before adding in the egg and a pinch of salt. Add in the flour and the knead the mixture until it forms a dough. If the dough sticks to your fingers add more flour.
- Add a pinch of salt to a pot of water before placing the pot on the stove over a burner turned to a high heat.
- While waiting for the water to boil, roll the dough into long, thick rolls about the width of a thumb. Chop each roll into 1-inch pieces and put a shallow indent in each.

- Place the gnocchi in the water using a slotted spoon. When they start to float they are ready to be removed. Place the finished gnocchi in a covered bowl to keep them warm.
- Add the oil to the skillet before placing it on the stove over a burner turned to a medium heat. Add in the garlic and let it cook about 4 minutes before adding the gnocchi and basil to the skillet and mix well. Cook about 2 minutes before adding in the pepper, lemon zest, lemon juice and salt.
- Top with cheese and basil prior to serving.

Chili

Total Prep & Cooking Time: 6 hours and 15 minutes
Yields: 8 Servings

What to Use
- Black pepper (as desired)
- Sea salt (as desired)
- Sweet potato puree (15 oz.)
- Red wine vinegar (2 tsp.)
- Chili powder (2 T)
- Celery (3 ribs diced fine)
- Onion (1 diced)
- Beef bone broth (2 c)
- Cloves (1 pinch ground)
- Cinnamon (1 pinch ground)
- Adobo sauce (1 T)
- Cumin (2 tsp. ground)
- Garlic (4 cloves minced)
- Grass-feed beef (2 lbs. ground)
- Avocado oil (1 T divided)
- Coconut aminos (2 tsp.)

What to Do
- Add the coconut oil to a skillet before placing it on the stove over a burner turned to a high heat. Add in .5 tsp. salt along with the ground beef and allow the meat to brown, using a spatula to break it up as you go. After about 5 minutes place the meat in your slow cooker.
- Reduce the burner heat to medium before adding in another tsp. of oil along with the onion, celery and garlic. Let everything cook for 5 minutes before adding in the chili powder, cinnamon, cloves and cumin. Let everything cook an additional 60 seconds while you stir. Add in the bone broth and let everything cook an additional 30 seconds before adding the contents of the skillet to the slow cooker.

- Add in the coconut aminos, vinegar, adobo sauce, sweet potato puree and season as desired.
- Cover the slow cooker and allow it to cook on a low heat for 6 hours.
- Top with lime wedges, scallions and sour cream prior to serving.

Instant Pot chicken

Total Prep & Cooking Time: 50 minutes
Yields: 4 Servings

What to Use
- Black pepper (as desired)
- Sea salt (as desired)
- Cilantro (.25 c)
- Ginger (1 in. chopped fine)
- Apple cider vinegar (2 T divided)
- Coconut aminos (.25 c + 1 T)
- Lime juice (1 lime)
- Garlic cloves (4)
- Salt (.5 tsp.)
- Raw honey (2 T)
- Mango (1 chunks)
- Green onion (1 sliced)
- Red onion (.5 chopped)
- Fish sauce (1 tsp)
- Chicken bone broth (.5 c)
- Chicken thighs (8 deboned)
- Cooking fat (1 T)

What to Do
- Heat your Instant Pot by pressing the sauté button before adding in the fat and allowing it to melt.
- Add in the chicken thighs with the skin facing down and allow it to cook for 3 minutes before flipping and allowing it to cook for 2 minutes more.
- Remove the chicken from the Instant Pot before adding in the garlic, mango and onion and allow them to cook about 5 minutes.
- Cancel the Instant Pot's sauté option before adding in the chicken, 1 T apple cider vinegar, honey, fish sauce, coconut aminos, chicken bone broth, lime juice, cilantro and ginger and mix well.

- Put the lid on the Instant Pot and select the poultry setting before choosing the option for high pressure which will automatically set a timer for 15 minutes.
- Manually release the pressure fully before removing the lid and removing the chicken from the Instant Pot.
- Add in the remaining apple cider vinegar and coconut aminos, along with a pinch of salt and return the Instant Pot to the sauté setting to allow the sauce to reduce until it reaches your desired level of thickness.
- Plate chicken and top with sauce and green onion prior to serving.

Cream soup

Total Prep & Cooking Time: 20 minutes
Yields: 4 Servings

What to Use
- Black pepper (as desired)
- Sea salt (as desired)
- Broccoli (2 c florets)
- Garlic (2 cloves chopped, peeled)
- Coconut milk (500 mL)
- Coconut flour (.25 c)
- Bay leaf (1)
- Rutabaga (2 c)
- Basil (.5 tsp. dried)
- Raw honey (1 tsp.)
- White onion (1 c diced)
- Beef bone broth (2 c)
- Grass-fed beef (1 lb.)
- Plantain (2 c)
- Cinnamon (.5 tsp.)
- Water (6 c)
- Carrots (1 c)

What to Do
- Add the water to your Instant Pot and use the sauté option to bring it to a boil before adding in your meat and letting it cook about 3 minutes.
- Drain the water and return the meat to the pot before adding in the bone broth as well as the vegetables before seasoning it with the cinnamon, herbs, salt and pepper and mixing well.
- Cover and seal the Instant Pot before setting it to 20 minutes.
- Use the quick release valve when time has elapsed and remove the vegetables and meat when it is safe to do so.

- Return the Instant Pot to the sauté setting before adding in the honey, coconut flour and coconut milk and mix well.
- Add in the broccoli and allow it to simmer before removing the cinnamon and bay leaf once the broccoli has finished cooking.
- Add all of the ingredients to a blender and blend well
- Season prior to serving.

Taco cups

Total Prep & Cooking Time: 90 minutes
Yields: 12 Servings

What to Use
- Black pepper (as desired)
- Sea salt (as desired)
- Chili powder (2 tsp.)
- Black beans (2 cans)
- Garlic powder (.25 tsp.)
- Onion (1 chopped fine)
- Avocado oil (3 T)
- Paprika (.5 tsp.)
- Coriander (1 tsp.)
- Palm shortening (.25 c)
- Coconut milk (.5 c room temp.)
- Cassava flour (1 c)
- Coconut aminos (1 tsp)
- Oregano (.5 tsp. dried)
- Water (.25 c)
- Taco cups (12)
- Ground cumin (2 tsp.)

What to Do
- Ensure your oven is heated to 425 degrees F.
- Prepare a muffin pan by turning it upside down and greasing it using 1 T avocado oil.
- In a mixing bowl, combine the water, palm shortening, cassava flour and coconut milk together and blend well.
- Form the resulting dough into 12 single oz. balls before rolling each ball out flat and placing them between 2 pieces of parchment paper
- Add the coconut oil to a skillet before placing it on the stove over a burner turned to a medium heat.

- Place the pieces of dough over the underside of the muffin cups to create bowls. Place the muffin tin in the oven for 20 minutes.
- Let the cups cool prior to filling.
- While the cups are baking, add the remaining oil to a skilling before placing it on top of a burner turned a medium heat. Add in the onions and let them cook for 2 minutes, stirring constantly. Add in the spice and coconut aminos and ensure the onions are well-coated before letting them cook an additional 60 seconds while stirring.
- Add the onions and black beans to the Instant Pot and season as desired. Close and seal the Instant Pot and turn it to a high pressure and cook 5 minutes. Let the pressure release naturally before seasoning as desired.
- Fill taco cups prior to serving.

Stuffed sausage

Total Prep & Cooking Time: 6 hours and 10 minutes
Yields: 5 Servings

What to Use
- Thyme (2 tsp. dried)
- Oregano (2 tsp. dried)
- Basil (2 tsp. dried)
- Garlic (.5 clove minced)
- White onion (1 small, diced)
- Cauliflower (.5 head processed to resemble rice)
- Bell peppers (5 seeded, peeled)
- Italian hot sausage (1 lb.)

What to Do
- Start by removing the top part of each pepper from the rest of the pepper. Save the top part of each pepper but remove and discard the seeds.
- Add the processed cauliflower to a mixing bowl before mixing in the onion, garlic, basil, thyme and oregano and combining well.
- Add the sausage to a skillet and place the skillet on the stove over a burner turned to a high/medium heat until it sears just enough to add to the favor.
- Add the sausage to the bowl of cauliflower and mix well.
- Add the results to the hollowed out peppers before placing each into your slow cooker and adding the tops of the peppers back in as well.
- Cover the slow cooker and let it cook on a low heat for 6 hours.
- Serve hot and enjoy.

Curry with Pineapple

Total Prep & Cooking Time: 6 hours and 5 minutes
Yields: 6 Servings

What to Use
- Black pepper (to taste)
- Salt (to taste)
- Lime juice (1 lime)
- Sweet potatoes (3 cups cubed)
- Carrot (3 chopped)
- Garlic (1 clove minced)
- Onion (.5 large diced)
- Garam masala (2 tsp.)
- Turmeric powder (.25 tsp.)
- Curry powder (.5 T)
- Vegetable stock (1 cup)
- Pumpkin puree (2 cups)
- Coconut milk (15 oz. unsweetened, full fat)

What to Do
- Add the pepper, salt, Garam masala, turmeric powder, curry powder, vegetable stock, pumpkin puree and coconut milk to the slow cooker before mixing well.
- Mix in the lime juice, sweet potatoes, carrots, garlic and onion and stir well.
- Cover the slow cooker and let it cook on a low heat for 6 hours.
- Serve hot over rice and enjoy.

Flap steak

Total Prep & Cooking Time: 4 hours and 30 minutes
Yields: 4 Servings

What to Use
- Black pepper (as needed)
- Salt (as needed)
- Coconut oil (2 T)
- Mango Salsa (as needed)
- Cumin (.5 tsp.)
- Coriander (.5 tsp.)
- Lime juice (1 T)
- White onion (.25 minced)
- Olive oil (.5 cups)
- Parsley (1 cup packed)
- Cilantro (1 cup packed)
- Flap steak (2 lbs. sliced thin)

What to Do
- In a food processor, combine .5 tsp. salt, cumin, coriander, lime juice, white onion, olive oil, parsley and cilantro and process well.
- Add the steak and half of the contents of a food processor to a resealable plastic bag before placing in the refrigerator to marinate for 4 hours.
- Let the steak sit at room temperature for half an hour before heating your grill to a high heat and cook the meat for approximately 2 minutes on each side.
- Top with the remaining marinade prior to serving.

Chowder

Total Prep & Cooking Time: 55 minutes
Yields: 5 Servings

What to Use
- Black pepper (as needed)
- Salt (as needed)
- Parsley (.25 cups chopped rough)
- Bay leaves (2)
- Chicken broth (6 cups)
- Thyme (1 tsp. dried)
- Oregano (1 tsp. dried)
- Smoked paprika (1 tsp.)
- Garlic powder (1 tsp.)
- Garlic (2 cloves chopped)
- Yellow onion (1 chopped)
- Celery (4 stalks diced)
- Carrots (2 diced, peeled)
- Shrimp (1 lb. deveined, peeled)
- Bacon (1.5 lbs.)
- Cauliflower (1 head florets, steamed, pureed)

What to Do
- Place a Dutch oven on the stove on top of a burner turned to a medium heat. Add in the bacon and let it cook until it reaches the desired level of crispness. Remove the bacon from the oven and add in the shrimp before seasoning as needed and cooking each side for 2 minutes.
- Add in the garlic, onion, celery and carrots and toss them in the bacon fat. After you can begin to see through the onion, mix in the salt, thyme, oregano, smoked paprika and garlic powder and stir for 60 seconds.
- Mix in the bay leaves as well as the chicken broth and the cauliflower. Mix in half of the cooked bacon and let it cook for 15 minutes.

- Take the bay leaves out of the mixture before adding in the parsley and pureeing everything in the Dutch Oven.
- Add in the shrimp and heat completely.
- Garnish with parsley, olive oil and bacon prior to serving.

Pot Roast

Total Prep & Cooking Time: 7 hours and 10 minutes
Yields: 6 Servings

What to Use-The Roast
- Parsley (1 T chopped)
- Garlic (3 cloves chopped)
- Onion (.5 sliced)
- Celery (2 stalks diced)
- Carrots (5 diced, peeled)
- Beef stock (1 cup)
- Coconut oil (1 T)
- Beef roast (3 lbs. fat removed)
- Allspice (.5 tsp. ground)
- Clove (.5 tsp. ground)
- Salt (1.5 tsp. ground)
- Cinnamon (2 tsp.)
- Coriander (1 T ground)
- Pepper (1 T)

What to Do
- Combine the allspice, clove, salt, cinnamon, coriander and pepper together and spread it over the meat.
- Place a skillet on the stove over a burner with the heat turned to medium before adding the coconut oil.
- Place the roast in the skillet and sear each side for a total of 10 minutes.
- Place the roast in the slow cooker along with the celery, garlic, onion and carrots.
- Add in the broth and let the slow cooker cook at a low temperature for 7 hours.
- Add the parsley on top, serve and enjoy.

Salmon with Capers

Total Prep & Cooking Time: 30 minutes
Yields: 4 Servings

What to Use
- Olive oil (to taste)
- Salt (to taste)
- Pepper (to taste)
- Thyme (1 T crushed)
- Capers (1 T)
- Lemon (1 thinly sliced)
- Salmon (32 oz.)

What to Do
- Cover a baking sheet with a rim in parchment paper.
- Put the salmon onto the baking sheet so that its skin touches the baking sheet.
- Add salt and pepper to the fish as you prefer before topping the fish with the caper, thyme and lemon.
- Place the fish in a cold oven, set the oven at 400 degrees Fahrenheit and let the fish cook for 25 minutes.
- Serve hot and enjoy.

Squash and Thai Curry

Total Prep & Cooking Time: 30 minutes
Yields: 4 Servings

What to Use
- Cauliflower rice (preparation details described below)
- Cilantro (.25 cups chopped)
- Lime juice (2 tsp.)
- Acorn Squash (1 peeled, seeded and cubed)
- Coconut aminos (1 T)
- Coconut milk (14 oz. can)
- Red curry paste (3 T)
- Ginger (1-inch peeled, minced)
- Garlic (4 cloves minced)
- Bell pepper (1 sliced)
- Salt (1 T)
- Onion (1 diced)
- Coconut oil (1 T)

What to Do
- Place a large pan on a burner which has been turned to a medium heat.
- Add in the coconut oil and the onion and let it cook for 6 minutes, be sure to stir.
- Mix in the salt, ginger, garlic and bell pepper and let cook for 60 seconds.
- Mix in the curry paste and let cook for an additional 60 seconds.
- Mix in the coconut aminos and milk before bringing the pan to a simmer.
- Mix in the squash and let the pan simmer for 20 minutes or until the squash has begun to grow tender.
- Take the pan from the heat, mix in the lime juice.
- Serve with cauliflower rice.

Chicken and blackberry mustard

Total Prep & Cooking Time: 20 minutes
Yields: 4 Servings

What to Use
- Blackberries (1 cup chopped)
- Mustard (1.5 T)
- Honey (2 tsp.)
- Chicken tenders (1 lb. halved)
- Salt (.5 tsp.)
- Black pepper (.25 tsp.)
- Cornmeal (3 T)
- Coconut oil (3 T)

What to Do
- Season the chicken as desired before adding it to a bowl of the cornmeal and coating well.
- Add the coconut oil to the skillet before adding the skillet to a burner turned to a high/medium heat.
- After the oil has melted, lower the heat to medium and add in the chicken and let each side cook for about 4 minutes. The internal temperature should read 165 degrees Fahrenheit.
- Remove the tenders from the stove and let them cool for a few minutes prior to serving.
- Add the mustard, honey and berries together, max and mix well.
- Serve with the chicken and enjoy.

Fish sandwich

Total Prep & Cooking Time: 20 minutes
Yields: 4 Servings

What to Use
- Salmon fillet (1 lb. quartered)
- Cajun seasoning (2 tsp.)
- Avocado (1 pitted, peeled)
- Mayonnaise (2 T)
- White rolls (4)
- Arugula (1 cup)
- Red onion (.5 cups sliced thin)
- Coconut oil (2 T)

What to Do
- Coat the grill in coconut oil before ensuring it is heated to a high heat.
- Coat the fish using the seasoning before adding it to the grill and let it cook for approximately 3 minutes on each side.
- Mash the avocado before mixing it with the mayonnaise and spreading on the rolls prior to serving.
- Season as required, serve hot and enjoy.

Chicken Pesto

Total Prep & Cooking Time: 45 minutes
Yields: 4 Servings

What to Use
- Black pepper (as desired)
- Sea salt (as desired)
- Olive oil (4 T)
- Leafy greens (5.3 oz.)
- Garlic (1 clove chopped fine)
- Feta cheese (8 oz. diced)
- Olives (8 T pitted)
- Heavy whipping cream (1.5 c)
- Green pesto (3 oz.)
- Butter (2 oz.)
- Chicken thighs (1.5 lbs.)

What to do
- Ensure your oven is heated to 400F.
- Cut the chicken into pieces before seasoning as desired and frying until it reaches an internal temperature of 165F.
- In a small mixing bowl, combine the heavy cream and the pesto.
- Add the chicken to a baking dish before adding in the garlic, feta cheese and olives and topping everything with the pesto mixture.
- Place the dish in the oven and let it cook for 30 minutes.

Meat Pie

Total Prep & Cooking Time: 15 minutes
Yields: 4 Servings

What to Use-Filling
- Water (.5 c)
- Dried oregano (1 T)
- Sea salt (as desired)
- Black pepper (as desired)
- Ground lamb (1.3 lbs.)
- Olive oil (2 T)
- Garlic (1 clove chopped fine)
- Yellow onion (.5 chopped fine)

What to Use-Crust
- Water (4 T)
- Egg (1 large, organic)
- Coconut oil (3 T)
- Salt (1 pinch)
- Baking powder (1 tsp.)
- Psyllium husk powder (1 T)
- Coconut powder (4 T)
- Almond flour (.75 c)

What to Use-Toppings
- Shredded cheese (7 oz.)
- Cottage cheese (8 oz.)

What to do
- Ensure your oven is heated to 350F.
- Add the olive oil to a skillet before placing it on the stove over a burned turned to a high/medium heat. Add in the garlic along with the onion and let them fry for 3 minutes or until they have softened.
- Add in the ground beef, basil and oregano and season as desired before adding in the tomato paste as well as

the water. Reduce the heat and let everything simmer 20 minutes. While this is taking place, make the crust.

- Combine the dough ingredients using a food processor and process until the results form a ball. The same effect can be achieved by hand mixing with a fork.
- Line greased 10-inch springform pan before spreading in the dough.
- Bake the crust for 15 minutes before removing it and adding in the filling.
- Mix together the shredded cheese and cottage cheese and add this on top.
- Bake 30 minutes and let sit 5 minutes prior to baking.

Turkey Wings

Total Prep & Cooking Time: 30 minutes
Yields: 4 Servings

What to Use
- Chopped thyme (1 bunch)
- Orange juice (1 c.)
- Chopped yellow onion (1)
- Pepper
- Salt
- Walnuts (1 c.)
- Dried cranberries (1.5 c.)
- Olive oil (2 Tbsp.)
- Coconut oil (2 T melted)
- Turkey wings (4)

What to Do
- Set your Instant Pot on Sauté mode and add the oil and ghee. When these are warm, add the pepper, salt, and turkey wings. Let the wings heat up on all sides.
- Add the thyme, cranberries, walnuts, and onion. Stir these around and cook for two minutes.
- Add the orange juice and then cover up the pot. Cook these on High for 20 minutes.
- Divide up the wings between a few plates and keep them warm.
- Set the pot to Simmer mode and cook your cranberry mix for another 5 minutes. Drizzle this on the turkey wings and serve.

Butternut and Chard Soup

Total Prep & Cooking Time: 30 minutes
Yields: 6 Servings

What to Use
- Coconut cream (1 c.)
- Minced garlic cloves (4)
- Cubed butternut squash (2 c.)
- Hopped Swiss chard (4 c.)
- Chopped rosemary (1 tsp.)
- Pepper
- Salt
- Chicken stock (8 c.)
- Thyme sprigs (4)
- Chopped celery stalks (3)
- Chopped carrots (3)
- Chopped yellow onion (1)
- Olive oil (1 Tbsp.)

What to Do
- Set the Instant Pot to Sauté mode before adding the oil. Add the celery, onion, and carrots.
- After those are warm, add the rosemary, garlic, butternut squash, pepper, salt, chicken stock, and thyme. Stir and cook this on a high setting for 18 minutes.
- Discard the thyme and add the coconut cream and Swiss chard. Warm up before serving.

Garlic Pot Roast

Total Prep & Cooking Time: 5 hours and 10 minutes
Yields: 8 Servings

What to Use
- Salt (as needed)
- Pepper (as needed)
- Beef stock (.75 cups)
- Garlic (1 tsp. minced0
- Bacon (6 slices, crumbled cooked)
- Beef shoulder (3 lbs.)

What to do
- Add the roast to the slow cooker and season as desired before topping with bacon and minced garlic.
- Add in the beef stock and set the slow cooker, covered, to high and let everything sit for 5 hours until the meat has reached its desired level of tenderness.

Meatballs

Total Prep & Cooking Time: 40 minutes
Yields: 3 Servings

What to Use
- Coconut oil (2 T)
- Pepper (as desired)
- Salt (as desired)
- Oregano (1 T)
- White onion (2 T diced)
- Garlic (2 T minced)
- Bacon (9 slices)
- Italian sausage (1 lb.)

What to Do
- Start by making sure your oven is heated to 375F.
- Cover a baking sheet using aluminum foil.
- Place a skillet on top of a burner that has been turned to a high/medium heat before adding in the coconut oil and the sausage and letting it brown.
- Add all of the ingredients, save the bacon to a mixing bowl and combine thoroughly.
- Form the results into 9 meatballs and wrap a slice of bacon around each before placing them on the baking sheet. Place the baking sheet in the oven for 30 minutes or until the bacon is well-cooked.
- Let cool 5 minutes prior to serving.

Sliders

Total Prep & Cooking Time: 45 minutes
Yields: 6 Servings

What to Use
- Water (.25 c)
- Heavy cream (.25 c)
- Salt (.5 tsp.)
- Garlic powder (.5 tsp.)
- Cheddar cheese (4 oz.)
- Butter (2 oz. unsalted)
- Carbquik (2 c)
- Hamburger (1 lb.)
- Cheddar cheese (6 slices)

What to Do
- Start by making sure your oven is heated to 450F.
- In a mixing bowl, add in the Carbquick before adding in the butter and mixing until the results start to form a dough.
- Add in the garlic powder, cheese and salt and mix well before adding in the liquid ingredients and mixing to form a dough.
- Form the dough into 6 equal sections and place them onto a prepared baking sheet.
- Place the baking sheet in the oven for 8 minutes until the biscuits are golden brown.
- While the biscuits are baking, place the hamburger into a skillet and place the skillet on top of a burner turned to a high/medium heat. As the meat browns, form it into small patties.
- Slice the biscuits in half, and a hamburger patty and slice of cheese to each.

Burger with egg

Total Prep & Cooking Time: 30 minutes
Yields: 3 Servings

What to Use
- Cheddar cheese (8 oz.)
- Worcestershire sauce (to taste)
- Onion powder (.5 tsp.)
- Garlic powder (.5 tsp.)
- Egg (2)
- Ground beef (1.5 lbs.)
- Coconut oil (2 T)
- Bacon (4 strips)

What to Do
- In a mixing bowl, combine the eggs and beef and mix well before adding in the spices and combining thoroughly.
- Break the results down into 1.5 oz. patties before topping each patty with .5 oz. of cheese.
- Combine every 2 patties into a single burger.
- Add the coconut oil to a pan before placing the pan on the stove on top of a burner turned to a high/medium heat. Add in one of the patties and cook each side for approximately 2 minutes or until it reaches your desired level of doneness.
- In a separate frying pan, add in the bacon before placing it on top of a burner turned to a high/medium heat and cook until crispy.
- Top each patty with bacon prior to serving.

Chapter 6: Snack Recipes

Stuffed poblano peppers

Total Prep & Cooking Time: 4 hours and 5 minutes
Yields: 4 Servings

What to Use
- Salt (as needed)
- Pepper (as needed)
- Onion (1 T chopped)
- Ground beef (.3 lbs.)
- Cauliflower (.3 c chopped fine)
- Poblano pepper (1)

What to Do
- Slice the poblano pepper in two and remove all of the seeds before setting it aside.
- Place the onion and the ground beef in a skillet before placing the skillet on the stove over a burner turned to a high/medium heat and cook for approximately 5 minutes. Stir regularly to ensure the ground beef browns fully.
- Add the results to the poblano halves.
- Add the tomato juice to the slow cooker before placing the stuffed peppers on top.
- Adjust the slow cooker temperature to low and leave it be, covered for about 4 hours.

Hummus

Total Prep & Cooking Time: 120 minutes
Yields: 18 Servings

What to Use
- Black pepper (as desired)
- Sea salt (as desired)
- Olive oil (2 T)
- Garlic (1 clove chopped)
- Lemon juice (1 lemon)
- Lemon zest (.5 lemons)
- Cumin (.25 tsp.)
- Tahini (.3 c)
- Garbanzo beans (.5 lbs.)
- Garlic powder (.5 tsp.)
- Water (3.5 c)

What to Do
- Add the salt, beans, garlic powder and water to the Instant Pot and mix well. Secure the lid, select high pressure and cook on manual mode for 1 hour.
- Wait for the pressure to decrease naturally before draining the beans while retaining the cooking liquid to use when making the hummus.
- Wait for the beans to cool enough to handle before placing them, .5 c cooking liquid, cumin, salt, olive oil, pepper, lemon zest, lemon juice and tahini in a food processor and process well.
- Check the hummus consistency and add more cooking liquid as needed.

Mashed Squash

Total Prep & Cooking Time: 25 minutes
Yields: 4 Servings

What to Use
- Black pepper (as desired)
- Sea salt (as desired)
- Brown sugar (2 T)
- Coconut oil (2 T)
- Nutmeg (.5 tsp. grated)
- Baking soda (.25 tsp.)
- Kosher salt (1 tsp.)
- Water (.5 c)
- Acorn squash (2 seeded, halved, trimmed)

What to Do
- Add the squash, baking soda and salt to a pressure.
- Add in the pressure cooker cooking rack along with .5 c water along with layers of squash.
- Secure the lid and turn the pressure to high, on a high temperature and allow the squash to cook about 20 minutes. Quick release the pressure and remove the squash from the cooker and place it in a large bowl.
- Scrape the squash flesh into the bowl before adding in the brown sugar, nutmeg and coconut oil.
- Mash the sweet potato using a potato masher. Check the flavor and season as desired prior to serving.

Pesto with parsley and cilantro

Total Prep & Cooking Time: 20 minutes
Yields: 4 Servings

What to Use
- Parsley (1 c)
- Lemon juice (.5 lemon)
- Cilantro (1 c packed loosely)
- Almonds (2 T sliced, blanched)
- Extra-virgin olive oil (.25 c)
- Salt (.5 tsp.)

What to Do
- Add half the olive oil, salt, cilantro, parsley, almonds and lemon juice to a blender and pulse to blend.
- Lower the blender speed and add the rest of the olive oil slowly. Blend until the pesto reaches your desired consistency.

Sprout chips

Total Prep & Cooking Time: 20 minutes
Yields: 2 Servings

What to Use
- Black pepper (as desired)
- Sea salt (as desired)
- Lemon zest (as desired)
- Coconut oil (2 T melted)
- Brussel sprout leaves (2 c)

What to Do
- Ensure your oven is heated to 350 degrees F.
- Coat the leaves using the coconut oil before seasoning as desired and place them on a baking sheet that has been prepared using parchment paper. Ensure the leaves lay flat in a single layer when you are finished.
- Place the baking sheet in the oven and let the leaves cook about 10 minutes or until the leaves are brown but crispy on the edges.

Cabbage wedges

Total Prep & Cooking Time: 30 minutes
Yields: 6 Servings

What to Use
- Black pepper (as desired)
- Sea salt (as desired)
- Avocado oil (.5 T)
- Cabbage wedges (1 head of cabbage)
- Lemon wedges (2 lemons)

What to Do
- Ensure your oven is heated to 450 degrees F.
- Place the cabbage on a baking sheet before brushing each wedge with oil to prevent it from burning. Try to keep everything covered evenly for the best result. Leave room between the wedges to ensure they get nice and crispy in the oven.
- Season as desired before placing the baking sheet in the oven for about 15 minutes. Remove the baking sheet, flip the wedges and return the baking sheet to the oven for an additional 10 minutes. You will know they are ready when the edges are crisp but the insides are still tender.
- Garnish with lemon.

Mashed cauliflower

Total Prep & Cooking Time: 20 minutes
Yields: 4 Servings

What to Use
- Black pepper (as desired)
- Sea salt (as desired)
- Coconut oil (2 T)
- Cauliflower (2 lbs. florets)
- Romano cheese (.5 c)
- Rosemary (2 tsp. dried)
- Chives (to taste)

What to Do
- Add .25 in. water to a frying pan before placing it on the stove over a burner turned to a high heat. Mix in .5 tsp. salt along with the cauliflower florets.
- Cover the pan and allow the cauliflower to steam for about 3 minutes if you like it crisp and 8 minutes if you prefer it soft.
- Drain the cauliflower and add it to a bowl before using a potato masher to mash them along with the coconut oil.
- Add the cheese and any seasonings prior to serving.

Oven fries

Total Prep & Cooking Time: 40 minutes
Yields: 8 Servings

What to Use
- Black pepper (as desired)
- Sea salt (as desired)
- Coconut oil (3 T)
- Sweet potatoes (2 striped)
- Garlic powder (2 tsp.)
- Grainy mustard (3 T)
- Purple carrots (halved, quartered)

What to Do
- Pace two baking sheets in the oven and ensure your oven is heated to 450 degrees F.
- Add the sweet potatoes and carrots to a bowl before coating well using the coconut oil and topping with black pepper, salt and garlic. Add the results evenly in single layers to the two baking sheets.
- Bake about 15 minutes before removing the baking sheets from the oven and tossing the fries to ensure they cook evenly. Return the baking sheets to the oven and cook an additional 15 minutes.
- While the fries are cooking add the pepper, sour cream and mustard to a small bowl and mix well.
- Serve fries with a side of dip.

Basil Pesto

Total Prep & Cooking Time: 20 minutes
Yields: 4 Servings

What to Use
- Sea salt (as desired)
- Coconut oil (.5 c)
- Parmesan cheese (.5 c grated)
- Garlic (2 cloves)
- Basil (2 c)

What to Do
- Add all of the ingredients, along with half of the coconut oil to a blender and pulse to blend.
- Lower the speed of the blender and slowly add the remaining oil in and blend until it reaches your desired texture.

Sage pesto

Total Prep & Cooking Time: 20 minutes
Yields: 4 Servings

What to Use
- Black pepper (as desired)
- Sea salt (as desired)
- Extra-virgin olive oil (.25 c)
- Garlic (1 clove minced)
- Sage leaves (1 c)

What to Do
- Add all of the ingredients, along with half of the coconut oil to a blender and pulse to blend.
- Lower the speed of the blender and slowly add the remaining oil in and blend until it reaches your desired texture.

Braised carrots with kale

Total Prep & Cooking Time: 30 minutes
Yields: 2 Servings

What to Use
- Black pepper (as desired)
- Sea salt (as desired)
- Onion (1 sliced thin)
- Chicken bone broth (.5 c)
- Coconut oil (1 T)
- Balsamic vinegar (1 T)
- Garlic (5 cloves chopped, peeled)
- Carrots (3 sliced)
- Kale (10 oz. chopped rough)

What to Do
- Set your Instant Pot to a medium heat and activate the sauté option before adding in your coconut oil. Once it has melted, add in the carrots and onions and let them cook about 5 minutes before adding in the garlic and cooking an additional 30 seconds. Add in the kale, broth and seasonings and mix well.
- Change the Instant Pot setting to manual and set the pot to cook 5 minutes. Secure the lid and allow the pressure to decrease naturally for about 10 minutes before activating the quick release valve.
- Remove the lid from the Instant Pot before adding in the vinegar and mixing well.
- Top with red pepper flakes for a bit of spice.

Beef bone broth

Total Prep & Cooking Time: 185 minutes
Yields: 16 Servings

What to Use
- Purified water (4 quarts)
- Apple cider vinegar (2 T)
- Salt (2 tsp.)
- Parsley (2 tsp. dried, crushed)
- Garlic (1 clove crushed)
- Ginger (1 tsp.)
- Lemon rind (2 tsp. ground)
- Yellow onions (2 chopped)
- Carrots (4 chopped)
- Celery (3 stalks chopped)
- Bouquet garni (1 tied with cooking twine)
- Meaty ribs (3 lbs.)
- Bone marrow (2 lbs.)
- Knucklebones (2 lbs.)

What to Do
- Roast the bones prior to making a stock for the best results.
- Add the knuckle bones, bone marrow, meaty ribs, bouquet garni, celery, carrots, yellow onions, lemon rind, ginger, apple cider vinegar and garlic to a large stockpot.
- Add in the water and let everything sit for 30 minutes to give the apple cider vinegar time to do its thing.
- Add the pot to the stove over a burner turned to a high heat before letting it boil. Reduce the heat and allow the pot to simmer for 180 minutes.
- 10 minutes before the stock has finished cooking, add in the salt as well as the parsley.

- Strain the stock prior to cooling or serving and save the results for another meal. Remember, fattier stocks will need a sturdy wire strainer.

Cajun Greens

Total Prep & Cooking Time: 35 minutes
Yields: 4 Servings

What to Use
- Black pepper (as desired)
- Sea salt (as desired)
- Onion (1 c chopped)
- Turnip (1 c chopped)
- Mustard (1 c chopped)
- Kale (1 c chopped)
- Collard greens (1 c chopped)
- Spinach (1 c chopped)
- Bacon fat (1 T)
- Garlic (2 cloves crushed)
- Ham (1 lb. cooked, chunked,
- Chicken bone broth (.5 c)

What to Do
- Add all of the ingredients to your Instant Pot, secure the lid, set the timer for 20 minutes and select the manual option after choosing high pressure.
- Allow the pressure to release manually for 10 minutes before venting the rest.
- Mix results together for flavor and serve.

Chickpea trail mix

Total Prep & Cooking Time: 17 minutes
Yields: 5 Servings

What to Use
- Black pepper (as desired)
- Sea salt (as desired)
- Cajun season (1 T)
- Ginger (1-inch ground)
- Cashews (.5 c)
- Chickpeas (1 c)
- Coconut oil (2 T)
- Raw honey (.5 c)
- Mango (6 oz. dried)
- Water (1 T)
- Almonds (1 c)
- Pecans (1.5 c halved)

What to Do
- Ensure your oven is heated to 375 degrees F.
- Add all of the ingredients save the coconut oil to your Instant Pot and mix well.
- Turn the Instant Pot to sauté and coat everything in the coconut oil and honey. After it has sautéed for a few minutes if it seems to thick or sticky add in the extra 1 T of water.
- Turn the pressure cooker to the manual setting and a high pressure and let it cook for 10 minutes, using the quick release pressure valve at that time.
- Spread the results on a baking sheet lined with parchment paper and place the baking sheet in the oven for 5 minutes, remove the baking sheet, toss the nuts and turn the sheet and return it to the oven for an additional few minutes, taking care not to burn the nuts.

- Remove the baking sheet from the oven and allow it to cool before adding in the mango. Pour the trail mix into an airtight container and shake well to combine.

Steamed Artichokes

Total Prep & Cooking Time: 25 minutes
Yields: 2 Servings

What to Use
- Black pepper (as desired)
- Sea salt (as desired)
- Lemon wedge (1)
- Artichoke (2)
- Water (1 c)

What to Do
- Rinse the artichokes before removing any damaged leaves as well as the stems using a sharp knife. From there, remove roughly the top third of the artichoke and then rub it with a lemon wedge to prevent it from browning in the heat.
- Set the basket in your Instant Pot before adding in your artichoke and the water. Seal the Instant Pot and set it to a high pressure in manual mode. The size of your artichoke will determine the cooking time with small artichokes cooking for 5 minutes, medium artichokes cooking for 10 minutes and large artichokes cooking for 15 minutes.
- All the pressure to release naturally for 10 minutes before using the manual release option.

Pork stew with pineapple

Total Prep & Cooking Time: 130 minutes
Yields: 6 Servings

What to Use
- Black pepper (as desired)
- Sea salt (as desired)
- Kumquat jam (2 T)
- Cloves (.5 tsp. ground)
- Bay leaf (1)
- Garlic (2 cloves chopped)
- Pineapple chunks (1 c)
- Turmeric powder (.5 tsp.)
- Cinnamon (1 tsp.)
- Cassava flour (.25 c)
- Ginger powder (.5 tsp.)
- Pork (2 lb. cubed)
- Coconut aminos (1 T)
- Bacon fat (2 T)
- Chard (1 bunch)
- Onion (1 wedged)
- Pork bone broth (1 c)

What to Do
- Turn your Instant Pot to Sauté and allow it to heat fully before adding in the fat and the onions and letting them cook about 5 minutes before adding in the garlic and letting it cook an additional 3 minutes before removing the garlic and onions from the Instant Pot and setting them aside.
- Add in some coconut oil if needed before adding in the porn and letting it brown. Return the garlic and onion to the pot before adding in the kumquat jam, cinnamon and bay leaf.

- Seal the Instant Pot and select the Stew option to set the timer for 35 minutes. When time is up, use the quick release option.
- Remove the lit and adjust the setting to sauté once more before adding in the chard.
- Discard the bay leaf and season as desired prior to serving.

Chicken bone broth

Total Prep & Cooking Time: 48 hours
Yields: 8 cups

What to Use
- 3 chicken carcasses
- 1 tablespoon of apple cider vinegar
- 1 bay leaf
- 2 onions
- 1 clove of garlic
- 2 tablespoons of peppercorns
- 3 celery stalks
- 3 carrots
- Parsley
- Thyme

What to Do
- Assemble all of the ingredients and place them in the crockpot (a 6-quart crockpot will hold all of the items plus the 2.5 quarts of water required).
- Set the crockpot on a low setting and cook for 24 to 48 hours.
- If you are interested in straining out the excess fat pour the contents through a wire strainer before cooling and storing.
- Note on storing, if your broth doesn't gel as discussed it is most likely because you added to much water, cut back next time to increase the nutritional value per cup.

Fishbone broth

Total Prep & Cooking Time: 24 hours
Yields: 8 cups

What's to Use
- Sea salt (to taste)
- Fish bones (2 lbs.)
- Apple Cider Vinegar (1 T)
- Water (3 quarts)

What to Do
- Place all of the items in a crockpot (6-quart or more)
- Place the crockpot on a low setting for about 24 hours, during this period foam will rise to the top which you want to remove as it contains impurities.
- When finished strain the broth with a wire strainer
- Cool and store

Turkey Bone Broth

Total Prep & Cooking Time: 48 hours
Yields: 8 cups

What to Use
- 1 large turkey carcass
- 1 tbsp. of apple cider vinegar
- 2 tbsps. of black pepper
- 2 leaves of bay
- 2 stalks of celery (2-inch pieces)
- 1 clove of garlic (halved)
- 1 onion (quartered)
- 1 leek (2-inch pieces)
- 2 carrots (2-inch pieces)

What to Do
1. Assemble all of the ingredients and place them in the crockpot (a 6-quart crockpot will hold all of the items plus the 2.5 quarts of water required).
2. Set the crockpot on a low setting and cook for 24 to 48 hours.
3. If you are interested in straining out the excess fat pour the contents through a wire strainer before cooling and storing.

Jicama fries

Total Prep & Cooking Time: 70 minutes
Yields: 4 Servings

What to Use
- Black pepper (as desired)
- Sea salt (as desired)
- Paprika (1 dash)
- Chili powder (1 tsp.)
- Garlic powder (.5 tsp.)
- Onion powder (.5 tsp.)
- Coconut oil (3 T)
- Jicama (1 lb.)

What to Do
- Ensure your oven is heated to 400 degrees F.
- Peel and slice the jicama so that the end result resembles a bowl of French fries.
- Add the jicama to a pot and fill it with water and a pinch of salt before placing it on the stove over a burner turned to a high heat. Allow the jicama to boil for about 15 minutes before removing from the pot and patting dry.
- Place the jicama on a baking sheet in an even layer and coat with the coconut oil.
- Combine the salt, pepper, onion, garlic and chili powder and mix well before using the results to coat the fries.
- Place the baking sheet in the oven for 20 minutes, remove the baking sheet and flip the fries before returning the baking sheet to the oven for another 20 minutes.
- Let them cool about 5 minutes prior to serving.

Chapter 7: Dessert Recipes

Cassava

Total Prep & Cooking Time: 35 minutes
Yields: 4 Servings

What to Use
- Goat's milk kefir (1.25 c)
- Vanilla extract (.5 tsp.)
- Coconut oil (3 T)
- Cinnamon (1 tsp.)
- Sea salt (.25 tsp.)
- Nutmeg (1 pinch)
- Eggs (2)
- Baking powder (1 T)
- Water (.25 c)
- Monk's fruit sweetener (2 T)
- Cassava flour (1 c)

What to Do
- Place a nonstick griddle on the stove over a burner turned to a low/medium heat.
- In a small bowl, mix together the kefir, water, eggs and vanilla before adding in the coconut oil.
- In a separate bowl, combine the nutmeg, cinnamon, baking powder, sweetener, flour and sea salt and mix well.
- Combine the two bowls and whisk well until the ingredients are thoroughly combined.
- Scoop the batter onto the griddle in .25 c dollops. Cook about 2 minutes per side.
- Top with butter and cinnamon prior to serving.

Balsamic strawberry sauce

Total Prep & Cooking Time: 25 minutes
Yields: 2 Servings

What to Use
- Water (.25 c)
- Raw honey (.25 c)
- Frozen strawberries (16 oz.)
- Balsamic vinegar (2 T)

What to Do
- Add the water and strawberries to a saucepan before placing it on the stove over a burner turned to a low heat. Allow it to reduce and melt the strawberries while stirring, until it forms a glaze.
- In the same saucepan add in the honey and balsamic vinegar and cook an additional 15 minutes.
- Add the results to an immersion mixer and mix until smooth.
- Return the mixture to the saucepan and turn the burner to a medium heat to allow the sauce to thicken. Stir regularly until it reaches the desired consistency before pouring it into a mason jar and placing it in the refrigerator to cool.

Cake in a mug

Total Prep & Cooking Time: 3 minutes
Yields: 1 serving

What to Use
- Sea salt (1 pinch)
- Seasonal fruit (1 T)
- Tiger nut flour (1 T)
- Coconut flour (1 T)
- Coconut oil (2 T)
- Egg (1 beaten)
- Baking powder (.5 tsp.)
- Monk fruit sweetener (.5 tsp.)
- Vanilla (.5 tsp.)

What to Do
- In a mug that is microwave safe, combine the vanilla, salt, sweetener, baking powder, tiger nut flour, coconut flour and oil and mix well.
- Add in the egg and use a fork to beat the batter until it is smooth. Scrape down the sides and the bottom to ensure the cake doesn't stick. Finally, fold in the fruit.
- Add the mug to the microwave and let it cook for 90 seconds.
- Allow the cake to cool 60 seconds before removing it from the mug.

Lectin-free yogurt

Total Prep & Cooking Time: 25 minutes
Yields: 4 Servings

What to Use
- Black pepper (as desired)
- Sea salt (as desired)
- Coconut milk (27 oz.
- Probiotic capsules (2)
- Vanilla extract (1 tsp.)
- Raw honey (2 T)

What to Do
- Place the coconut milk in the refrigerator overnight to give the milk time to separate from the cream.
- Open the cans and scrape the cream into a bowl before adding in the probiotic capsules after breaking them open. Add in the vanilla and honey and blend thoroughly.
- Divide between an appropriate number of glass jars before placing each jar in your yogurt maker and following the relevant instructions. Allow the finished product to it at least 15 hours. The longer it is allowed to ferment, the sourer the end product will be.

Green Smoothie

Total Prep & Cooking Time: 15 minutes
Yields: 2 Servings

What to Use
- Mint leaves (2 T)
- Ginger root (1 T chopped)
- Banana (1 chopped)
- Avocado (.5)
- Lime juice (1 T)
- Chard (.5 c)
- Spinach (1 c)
- Kale (.5 c)
- Sea salt (1 pinch)
- Ice cubes (4)
- Sparkling water (16 fl. oz.)

What to Do
- Chill the sparkling water
- Add all of the ingredients to a blender and select the puree option before blending for one minute or until smooth. If the results are too thick to drink readily add additional sparkling water to thin as desired.

Chocolate cherry cupcakes

Total Prep & Cooking Time: 75 minutes
Yields: 18 Servings

What to Use
- Tart cherry juice (.25 c + .5 T)
- Erythritol (1 c + 1 T)
- Black cherries (1 lb.)
- Sea salt (1 pinch)
- Coconut oil (.25 c)
- Espresso (1 splash)
- Heavy whipping cream (1 c)
- Dark chocolate shavings (.25 c)
- Egg (1)
- Cocoa powder (.3 c)
- Lemon juice (1 T)
- Salt (.5 tsp.)
- Coconut oil (.25 c)
- Baking soda (.75 tsp.)
- Monk fruit sweetener (.5 c)
- Cassava flour (.75 c)
- Vanilla extract (.5 tsp)
- Coconut milk (.75 c)

What to Do
- Separate 20 cherries from the rest and set aside. Add the rest of the cherries to a large bowl before adding in .25 c tart cherry juice and allowing them to soak overnight.
- Ensure your oven is heated to 350 degrees F.
- Grease a large cupcake tin using coconut oil
- In a mixing bowl, combine the vinegar and coconut milk and let it sit for 10 minutes.
- Use a sieve to add the salt, cocoa powder, flour and baking soda together in a separate bowl.

- In a third bowl, combine the sweetener and the cream
  until blended well before adding in the eggs and
  combining thoroughly.
- Alternate between adding wet and dry ingredients to
  the milk and vinegar mixture, taking care to ensure
  everything is well-mixed.
- Add the resulting batter to the cupcake cups so that
  they are each about 75 percent full to give them room
  to expand as they bake.
- Add the cupcake tin to the oven for 20 minutes. You
  will know the cupcakes are done if you can stick a
  toothpick into the middle cupcake and pull it out
  clean.
- To make the filling, beat the butter in a mixing bowl
  until it is nice and creamy before adding in the salt,
  espresso and sweetener. Add in the cherry juice 1 T at
  a time to thin out the mixture as needed.
- Cut each cupcake in half before adding cherry juice
  and filling to each cupcake, along with one of the
  reserved cherries. Return the removed cupcake half to
  make a cupcake sandwich.
- Make the frosting by taking any remaining cherry
  juice and whipping it with vanilla and crema
  sweetener in a mixing bowl. Add the results to a
  pastry bag to decorate the cupcakes.

Instant Pot applesauce

Total Prep & Cooking Time: 30 minutes
Yields: 4 Servings

What to Use
- Apples (12 cored, diced)
- Apple cider (.5 c)

What to Do
- Place the apples in the Instant Pot before adding in the apple cider which will prevent the apples from getting too dry in the pot which will ultimately make it easier to make them into a sauce.
- Cut holes out of a large piece of parchment paper such that it will fit over the inner rim of the Instant Pot and place it on top of the apples to ensure they retain as much heat as possible.
- Seal the lid on the Instant Pot, set it to manual and set the time to 10 minutes. Allow the pressure to release naturally when the time is up.
- Using an immersion blender, blend the apples until they reach your desired consistency.
- Pour the applesauce into mason jars and cool prior to serving.

Strawberry shortcake

Total Prep & Cooking Time: 60 minutes
Yields: 8 Servings

What to Use
- Tiger nut flour (.3 c)
- Baking soda (.75 tsp.)
- Fine sea salt (.5 tsp.)
- Golden monk fruit (.25 c)
- Vanilla extract (.5 tsp.)
- Eggs (3)
- Coconut oil (8 T)
- Coconut cream (.5 c)
- Arrowroot starch (3 T)
- Lemon zest (.5 lemons)
- Coconut flour (.3 c)
- Strawberries (1 qt. sliced, hulled)
- Vanilla extract (.5 tsp.)
- Raw honey (1 T)
- Heavy cream (1 c)

What to Do
- Ensure your oven is heated to 350 degrees F.
- Grease a round cake pan (8 in.) using coconut oil before lining it with parchment paper. Finally, grease it again before coating the grease in a light sprinkling of flour.
- With the help of a stand mixer, combine the coconut oil, coconut cream and sweeteners before adding in the eggs, vanilla extract and lemon zest and blending well to combine thoroughly.
- In a separate bowl, combine the sea salt, tiger nut flour, arrowroot starch, coconut flour and baking soda and mix well before adding it to the mixer mixture and blending on a low speed until smooth.

- Add the batter to the baking pan, ensuring the top is smooth and bubble free. Tapping the pan on the counter will help to release trapped air bubbles and settle the batter.
- Place the pan in the oven for about 25 minutes or until you can stick a knife into the center of the cake and pull it out clean.
- Remove the cake from the oven and allow it to cool for 30 minutes before removing it from the pan and placing it on a rack where you are to allow it to continue to cool until it reaches room temperature.
- With the help of the stand mixer, combine the cream, honey and vanilla extract at high speed until peaks begin to form.
- Frost the cake prior to serving.

Blueberry dessert

Total Prep & Cooking Time: 60 minutes
Yields: 4 Servings

What to Use
- Whipping cream (8 oz.)
- Xylitol (3 T divided)
- Salt (1 pinch)
- Vanilla extract (.5 tsp.)
- Blueberries (2 c)
- Lemon (.5 zested, juiced)
- Heavy cream (1.3 c)

What to Do
- Add the salt, 1.5 c blueberries and 2 T xylitol into a boiler set to a medium heat and let everything heat until it begins to bubble. Reduce the temperature to low and stir constantly for 5 minutes.
- Remove the boiler from heat before adding in the rest of the blueberries, lemon zest and lemon juice and mix well before allowing the mixture to reach room temperature.
- While waiting for this to occur, combine the xylitol, vanilla and heavy whipping cream in a small bowl and whisk well to combine thoroughly. Continue whisking until it begins to form peaks before folding in the blueberry sauce gently.
- Divide into serving dishing and top with blueberries and chocolate shavings.

Mug gingerbread

Total Prep & Cooking Time: 15 minutes
Yields: 4 Servings

What to Use
- Cinnamon (.25 tsp.)
- Water (.5 T)
- Raw honey (2 tsp.)
- Tiger nut (1 T)
- Baking powder (.5 tsp.)
- Coconut flour (1 T)
- Coconut oil (1 T)
- Ground ginger (.5 tsp.)
- Apple cider vinegar (.5 tsp.)
- Cloves (1 pinch)
- Nutmeg (1 pinch)
- Allspice (1 pinch)
- Egg (1 beaten)

What to Do
- In a mug that is microwave safe, combine all the ingredients save the egg and mix well.
- Add in the egg and use a fork to beat the batter until it is smooth. Scrape down the sides and the bottom to ensure the cake doesn't stick. Finally, fold in the fruit.
- Add the mug to the microwave and let it cook for 90 seconds.
- Allow the cake to cool 60 seconds before removing it from the mug.

Ginger cake

Total Prep & Cooking Time: 60 minutes
Yields: 12 Servings

What to Use
- Sea salt (.25 tsp.)
- Coconut oil (.25 c softened)
- Pumpkin pie spice (2 tsp.)
- Ginger (.5 tsp. ground)
- Vanilla extract (2 tsp. divided)
- Baking soda (.75 tsp.)
- Almond flour (.3 c)
- Erythritol (.5 c)
- Cassava flour (.75 c)
- Eggs (2)
- Baking powder (.5 tsp.)
- Cream cheese (4 oz. softened)
- Confectioners erythritol (.75 c)

What to Do
- Ensure your oven is heated to 300 degrees F and your oven rack is set to the center of your oven.
- Grease a glass pan (9 x 13) with coconut oil.
- Combine the coconut milk and apple cider vinegar in a measuring cup and mix well before setting aside.
- In a mixing bowl, combine the salt, baking soda, ginger, flour and pumpkin pie spice and whisk well.
- In a separate bowl, beat the eggs with the coconut oil and sugar before adding in the vanilla and coconut milk and mixing well.
- Combine the two bowls and use a spatula to stir. The batter should be very thick.
- Add the cake batter to a greased pan and use a spatula to ensure it spreads easily. Tap the pan to remove any air bubbles.

- Place the pan in the oven for about 40 minutes. You will know its ready when you can stick a knife in the center and pull it out clean.
- For the icing, start by beating together the cream cheese and erythritol at a slow speed before adding in the vanilla extract and blending well. You will want the end result to be thin enough to spread with a knife but not so thin that it drips off the knife. If it is too thick to start you can thin it out by adding 1 T of water at a time until it reaches your desired thickness.
- Frost the cake and top with cinnamon.

Mint Pesto

Total Prep & Cooking Time: 20 minutes
Yields: 4 Servings

What to Use
- Sliced almonds (.25 c blancedo
- Coconut oil (3 T divided)
- Mint leaves (1 c packed loose)
- Raw honey (.25 c)

What to Do
- Add all of the ingredients save 2 T coconut oil to a blender and pulse well until thoroughly combined.
- Slowly add in the remaining coconut oil while blending at a slow speed. Continue blending until your desired texture is reached.

Peach cobbler

Total Prep & Cooking Time: 40 minutes
Yields: 4 Servings

What to Use
- Peaches (2 sliced thin)
- Baking soda (.25 tsp.)
- Baking powder (.25 tsp.)
- Fine sea salt (.25 tsp.)
- Cassava flour (.25 c)
- Goat's milk kefir (5 oz.)
- Liquid stevia (5 drops)
- Coconut flour (.25 c)
- Coconut oil (1 T)
- Vanilla extract (1 tsp.)
- Tapioca flour (.25 c)
- Egg (2)

What to Do
- Ensure your oven is heated to 350 degrees F.
- In a mixing bowl, beat the eggs, kefir, stevia and vanilla together and mix well before adding in the coconut oil and whisking steadily to prevent it from solidifying.
- Mix in the baking soda, baking powder, sea salt, cassava flour, tapioca flour and coconut flour and mix well. Whisk steadily until the batter is fully smooth.
- Add the results to a pie pan before placing half of the peaches into a single layer on top before seasoning with cinnamon.
- Place the pie tin in the oven for 30 minutes, you will know it is ready when you can stick a toothpick into the center of the pie and pull it out clean.
- Top with remaining peach slices prior to serving.

Conclusion

Thank you for making it through to the end of *Lectin-Free Cookbook: Delightful & Delicious Lectin-Free Recipes*, let's hope it was informative and able to provide you with all of the tools you need to achieve your goals, whatever it is that they may be. Just because you've finished this book doesn't mean there is nothing left to learn on the topic, expanding your horizons is the only way to find the mastery you seek.

When you are first making the transition to the lectin-free diet, it is important to always keep in mind that it isn't all or nothing. That is to say, just because you may find yourself in a situation where you aren't able to make a lectin-free choice, doesn't mean that you are somehow failing at the lectin-free diet. On the contrary, every single meal where you actively decrease the amount of lectin in your diet is a win and every meal where this doesn't happen is simply a chance to do better next time. As long as you don't let a single mistake turn into a prolonged binge of unhealthy foods full of lectin then there is nothing to hang your head about when you step out of line. Just remember, following the lectin-free diet is a marathon, not a sprint which means slow and steady will always win the race.

Finally, if you found this book useful in any way, a review on Amazon is always appreciated!

www.ingramcontent.com/pod-product-compliance
Lightning Source LLC
Chambersburg PA
CBHW070126260726
48658CB00001B/287